D0982402

THE
Anti-Inflammatory
Kitchen
COOKBOOK

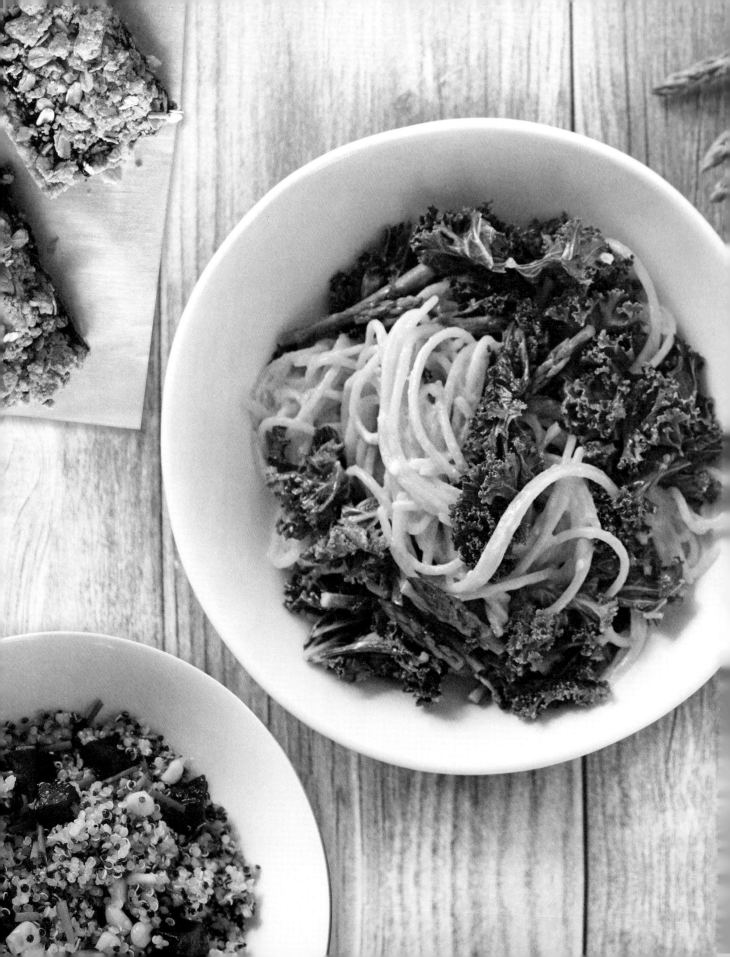

THE

Anti-Inflammatory
Kitchen

COOKBOOK

More Than 100 Healing, Low-Histamine,
Gluten-Free Recipes

Leslie Langevin, MS RD CD

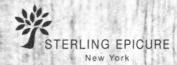

STERLING EPICURE
New York

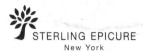

STERLING EPICURE
New York

An Imprint of Sterling Publishing Co., Inc.
1166 Avenue of the Americas
New York, NY 10036

ISBN 978-1-4549-3138-6

Distributed in Canada by Sterling Publishing Co., Inc.
c/o Canadian Manda Group, 664 Annette Street
Toronto, Ontario M6S 2C8, Canada
Distributed in the United Kingdom by GMC Distribution Services
Castle Place, 166 High Street, Lewes, East Sussex BN7 1XU, United Kingdom
Distributed in Australia by NewSouth Books
University of New South Wales, Sydney, NSW 2052, Australia

For information about custom editions, special sales, and premium and corporate purchases,
please contact Sterling Special Sales at 800-805-5489 or specialsales@sterlingpublishing.com.

Manufactured in Canada

2 4 6 8 10 9 7 5 3 1

sterlingpublishing.com

Interior design by Shannon Nicole Plunkett
Cover design by Elizabeth Lindy

CONTENTS

Preface

....

After a Christmas week full of work stress, family time, and celebration, I was looking forward to a nice, relaxing evening and a lovely glass of red wine. This particular wine came from a vineyard that my husband and I had visited years earlier, and we frequently enjoyed sipping it in our household. Except this time, just one sip left me feeling flushed and fatigued. After ten minutes, the side of my face started swelling, then a lump in my throat started to form—and grew bigger. I had no idea what was happening, so I called my physician. He said that I was going into anaphylactic shock and told me to go immediately to the nearest emergency room.

The harrowing ten-minute drive to the ER felt like an eternity. An inexplicable heart-pounding, crushing anxiety was making me shake and sweat. At the ER, my throat was closing tighter, barely allowing me to breathe. How could one sip of wine—that I had consumed before—trigger such a terrible reaction? The hospital staff pumped me full of antihistamines and steroids, and the doctors confirmed that I had experienced a severe allergic reaction. For the rest of the week, I felt terrible and out of sorts, suffering from lingering headaches, exhaustion, and brain fog.

Feeling a bit better, I returned home after a long day, looking forward to one of my favorite meals: a turkey burger with cheddar cheese and barbecue sauce served with maple-glazed carrots. That meal caused another severe reaction. Clearly my body had developed some kind of allergy, but how could I be allergic to what felt like everything, so severely, and all of a sudden? I thought critically, as a dietician, about what everything I had eaten in both instances had in common. Red wine, barbecue sauce, turkey burgers, and cheese all contain large amounts of histamine. Based on the results of my research and my professional knowledge, I identified which foods likely were causing my symptoms, then started a low-histamine diet the next day. In the year since then, I created many of the recipes that appear in this book.

My research revealed that I could have mast cell activation syndrome (MCAS). In less severe cases, it's called histamine intolerance, which is what happens when your body reacts adversely to the presence of too much histamine. Allergic reactions and the other symptoms associated with MCAS can be common and attributable to many other causes. Some of the symptoms, most of which I experienced, include clogged ears and sinuses, diarrhea, dizziness and feeling faint, eczema, flushed skin after eating, foggy thinking, heartburn, rapid heartbeat, tingling throat, and upset stomach—a complicated jumble indicating a variety of possible illnesses. It was unpleasant at best and completely debilitating at worst.

Luckily my diagnosis came very quickly. The histamine levels in my body likely had been increasing slowly over time. The headaches and stomach issues I had been experiencing before that glass of red wine and the trip to the ER seemed like the symptoms of everyday stress, but they were warning signs that my body was reaching a tipping point.

As a dietitian, I know first-hand that what you eat can make a difference in your health and how you feel. I decided to write this book to provide recipes that I developed during my own journey that can help other people. Whether you have a histamine intolerance, rheumatoid arthritis, interstitial cystitis, or inflammatory bowel disease, these anti-inflammatory recipes can help improve your daily life.

So let's get started.

Introduction

···

If such problems as chronic allergies, anxiety, brain fog, hives, fatigue, headaches, interstitial cystitis, irritable bowel syndrome, or pain have plagued you, there could be a simple solution. It's not another medication but rather a simple dietary change to an anti-inflammatory, low-histamine lifestyle. Changing your diet can help alleviate many different types of symptoms and improve your overall health. The recipes in this book will show you how to make real, homemade food in a short amount of time each day to help heal yourself and improve your health by reducing inflammation.

Real, fresh food can prove hard to find these days. Even when you make the effort to buy healthy, you often end up with food labeled "healthy" that actually contains unrecognizable, highly processed, non-nutritious ingredients. Swiss physician Theophrastus von Hohenheim (known as Paracelsus) receives credit for the concept that "the dose makes the poison," meaning that the only difference between medicine and poison is the amount consumed. Food is no different in that regard. It can be the strongest medicine or a slow poison.

In this book, we'll explore the science behind histamine intolerance, its related conditions, including mast cell activation syndrome (MCAS), and the diet that can help restore your health and well-being. The use of functional nutrition to help heal underpins this cookbook, but supplements and lifestyle are as important as the foods we put in our bodies, and we'll explore these in detail as well. This is not an extreme diet, however. I *love* food—the stuff you pull from the ground—the vivid colors, the smell of the earth, the knowledge that each bite is nourishing my body. The anti-inflammatory, low-histamine diet focuses on balance, moderation, and harnessing the powers of natural, everyday foods. It requires excluding high-histamine ingredients from your diet for a period of time, yes, but it's an elimination diet, which removes the top offenders for at least four weeks and then permits you to reintroduce those foods slowly back into your diet. It's rich in beans, fresh lean meat and fish, fruits, gluten-free whole grains, herbs, olive oil, seeds, and vegetables, and it's low in refined sugars, red meats, and processed foods. It's consistent with a Mediterranean diet, which has anti-inflammatory properties and can improve many health conditions, including the symptoms associated with histamine intolerance.

Before undertaking any special diet or taking any supplement, consult with your doctor to make sure it won't affect any medications that you may be taking or conditions that you may have.

HISTAMINE & INFLAMMATION

Histamine is a substance that the body releases from basophils, mast cells, and platelets in response to allergic reactions. It can derive from the amino acid histadine in high-protein foods and is found naturally in many aged and fermented foods. It works in the body by helping to stimulate gastric acid secretions in the stomach (which is why heartburn often results from excess histamine), controlling cell contraction and vasodilation (relaxing of blood vessels), and affecting blood pressure. Histamine clearly is helpful—except for when it proliferates either from the body releasing too much or not processing a surplus amount.

Histamine intolerance may occur in the body in a few ways. One is when enzymes responsible for breaking down histamine in the intestines and the rest of the body aren't functioning properly. The enzymes responsible for clearing histamine are called diamine oxidase (DAO) and histamine-N-methyltransferase (HNMT). Studies have shown that many individuals with inflammatory bowel disease (IBD) or irritable bowel syndrome (IBS) may have altered DAO or HNMT levels. Mast cell activation is when there is an increased number of mast cells, or they are more active and release uncontrolled amounts of histamine and inflammatory compounds. Our bodies release histamine during digestion and other normal processes, so it's impossible to suppress all histamine production, nor would we want to do that.

Mast Cells & Histamine Intolerance

Medical literature has recorded the effects of histamine intolerance for years. A study from the *American Journal of Clinical Nutrition* indicates that approximately 1 percent of the population has some degree of histamine intolerance. The full roster of symptoms includes acid reflux, allergic reaction, arrhythmia, asthma, brain fog, congestion, diarrhea, flushing of the skin, headache, hives, and hypotension. That's not a large percentage, but it still adds up to a lot of people. Many more people with a histamine sensitivity have allergies, asthma, chronic hives, IBS, and interstitial cystitis. A variety of factors can cause each of these symptoms, so people don't always realize that seemingly unrelated indicators may point to some level of histamine intolerance. This misunderstanding often results in treatment of the symptoms rather than the underlying problem.

Do you have any of the following symptoms?

- ☐ acid reflux
- ☐ allergies
- ☐ anxiety
- ☐ asthma
- ☑ chronic pain
- ☑ dermatitis or skin irritation, such as eczema
- ☐ dizziness on standing
- ☑ fatigue
- ☐ flushing (heat and redness usually in the face)
- ☑ excessive gas or diarrhea

- ☐ headaches or migraine
- ☐ hives or chronic hives
- ☐ interstitial cystitis
- ☑ irritable bowel syndrome
- ☐ itchy eyes
- ☐ low blood pressure
- ☐ nasal congestion
- ☐ rapid heart beat
- ☐ throat tightness or itching of lips, tongue or throat

If you do—and especially if you have more than one—you could benefit from a low-histamine, anti-inflammatory diet. Again, many of these commonly result from other health problems, so always consult with your physician to make sure that any new diet or change in your diet won't adversely affect any medications or existing medical conditions.

Why does this happen? Science still doesn't have a conclusive answer. Some environmental, lifestyle, medical, and genetic traits can increase your likelihood of developing histamine-related health problems, and we'll look at these traits and their causes in detail.

Potential causes of developing histamine intolerance:

- ☐ certain medications
- ☐ disruption of the microbiome, or the balance of bacteria in the gut
- ☐ extreme stress
- ☐ genetics
- ☐ impaired methylation. If your body isn't making enough HNMT (an enzyme) histamine can build up.
- ☐ nutrient deficiencies that impair your production of histamine-breakdown enzymes

- ☐ low diamine oxidase activity. DAO is another enzyme responsible for breaking down histamine. If your body doesn't have enough DAO, your histamine levels can increase.
- ☐ overactivation of mast cells, mast cell activation syndrome, or mastocytosis

Symptoms appear all over your body because histamine releases from the white blood cells called mast cells and basophils that exist all over the body. Mast cells are the immune cells that release pro-inflammatory molecules called cytokines, such as interleukin-8 (IL-8), tumor necrosis factor (TNF), and histamine. Basophils are white blood cells involved in inflammatory reactions in the body. Mast cells and basophils are important for your immune response to keep your body healthy, such as for fighting an infection. But in a person with histamine intolerance or mast cell activation, the surplus release of histamine increases inflammation or even triggers anaphylaxis. That's why a common link exists among inflammatory diseases, such as IBD, rheumatoid arthritis, certain forms of heart disease, and other histamine-related conditions.

HISTAMINE & INFLAMMATION-RELATED CONDITIONS

Let's look at some histamine-related conditions in more detail. When histamine is released in the body, so are inflammatory molecules, so it is likely that if you have a histamine-related condition, you also have a higher level of inflammation.

ALLERGIES & ASTHMA

The connection between histamine and inflammation forms the cornerstone of the understanding of allergies and asthma. Symptoms run the gamut from mild rhinitis (stuffy nose) to anaphylaxis. One study from the *American Journal of Clinical Nutrition* found that the ingestion of histamine-rich foods such as red wine increased the prevalence of allergy and asthma symptoms and proposed the cause as reduced HNMT and DAO activity.

The Mediterranean diet is an evidence based anti-inflammatory diet. It's rich in fruits, vegetables, whole grains, nuts and seeds, olive oil, and omega-3 fatty acids from fish—the base of the anti-inflammatory diet—and is low in processed foods, dairy, red meat, other meats, and sugar. Many studies, especially the 2013 PREDIMED study, have shown it to reduce inflammatory cytokine levels. An anti-inflammatory Mediterranean diet has shown promise in reducing nasal allergy symptoms, asthma, and allergic rhinitis. Researchers at the London National Heart and Lung Institute found that children who ate at least two servings of fresh fruits and vegetables daily had reduced incidence of allergic rhinitis. Eating nuts helped protect against wheezing in children with asthma, whereas greater intake of margarine increased wheezing and allergic rhinitis. The ISAAC study, which looked at 50,000 children from all over the world, found that the consumption of fish, vegetables, and fruit had an association with less wheezing and that hamburger consumption had a link to a higher prevalence of lifetime asthma. So eating anti-inflammatory whole foods, lots of fish, veggies, and fruit may offer protection against asthma and allergy symptoms.

ECZEMA & ATOPIC DERMATITIS

Eczema can occur from allergies or non-allergic inflammation. Research published by the *Journal of Allergy and Clinical Immunology* has shown that, due to genetic predisposition, many individuals with eczema may have a decreased ability to break down histamine because of low DAO levels. Further research from Charité Universitätsmedezin Berlin found that patients with eczema had increased symptoms after eating high-histamine foods. They also found an improvement in eczema symptoms by following a histamine-free diet. In a double-blind placebo study, patients with atopic dermatitis or eczema received either a placebo or an oral dose of histamine while following a histamine-free diet. A third of the group improved after following the histamine-free diet for only one week, and those who received oral histamine vs. placebo had an increase in symptoms showing the realtionship between histamine and eczema or atopic dermatitis.

HEADACHES & MIGRAINES

Evidence also supports that people who develop headaches or migraines may have a deficiency of the DAO enzyme, thereby decreasing the body's ability to break down histamine. Researchers from the University of British Columbia noted that frequent migraine triggers include alcohol (red wine), artificial sweeteners, caffeine, chocolate, dairy (aged cheese), monosodium glutamate, nitrates, and nitrites—all of which are high in histamine. Another group of allergists in Vienna found that low-histamine diets reduced headaches in a study group by 73 percent in only four weeks.

Chronic urticaria, or hives, is a presentation of itchy wheals or swelling of the skin that lasts for more than six weeks. Hives can result from an allergic reaction, but the majority of cases occur for no known reason. Researchers believe that this condition may develop from a defect in histamine metabolism, which causes the HNMT and DAO enzymes to work improperly. In one study in the *European Journal of Clinical Nutrition*, patients with chronic hives who followed a low-histamine and anti-allergen diet (no preservatives, no flavor additives, no food coloring) reported 30 percent remission, 30 percent partial remission, and 40 percent transient relapses. Following the diet for ten weeks allowed the patients' low DAO levels to increase and histamine levels to reduce to normal. Researchers in Germany also found that the symptoms of 75 percent of patients with chronic hives and gastrointestinal symptoms improved after following a low-histamine diet for just three weeks.

INTERSTITIAL CYSTITIS

Interstitial cystitis (IC) is a chronic inflammatory disease of the bladder that mast cells can directly affect, cause, or exacerbate, and IC occurs commonly in patients with mast cell activation and mastocytosis. Research has shown that patients with IC have increased levels of histamine in their urine, and in both human and animal studies the presence of histamine increased cystitis pain. Studies in the *Gynecology and Endocrinology* journal and researchers at Northwestern University found that an increase in mast cells may increase chronic pelvic pain. A separate study from researchers at the University of Iowa treated animals with IC with cromolyn sodium, a mast cell–stabilizing medication, which reversed bladder inflammation and IC symptoms. Quercetin, a bioflavonoid found in apples (page 15), may help stabilize mast cells and reduce IC symptoms. UCLA researchers provided quercetin supplements (500 mg twice a day) to patients with interstitial cystitis, who subsequently reported improvement in their IC symptoms.

IRRITABLE BOWEL SYNDROME (IBS) & IRRITABLE BOWEL DISEASE (IBD)

The microbiome—the combination of bacteria, yeast, and other microorganisms living in your digestive tract—represents an important piece of the puzzle for many histamine-intolerance cases. The type of bacteria present in your digestive system can determine how much DAO you produce and how effectively your body breaks down histamine. Research has shown that certain bacteria increase histamine production in the gut, namely *Lactobacillus bulgaricus*, *Lactobacillus casei*, *Lactobacillus delbrueckii*, and *Lactobacillus reuteri*. Having large colonies of these bacteria may prove problematic for your body because research has shown that people with IBS and IBD have elevated levels of histamine in their systems. Researchers continue to investigate the link between histamine and IBS, finding that high-histamine foods can trigger IBS symptoms. Patients commonly report diarrhea as a symptom of MCAS and histamine intolerance. Researchers from Sweden's Institute of Medicine noted that in one study about 50 percent of participants reported increased IBS symptoms when consuming high-histamine foods.

The Swiss Institute of Allergy and Asthma Research found that patients with IBD have elevated levels of mast cells, which release histamine and increase inflammation, and their more inflamed tissue contained more mast cells. The HNMT enzyme doesn't function efficiently in inflamed tissue, and DAO enzyme production also decreases, which causes increased histamine intolerance and GI symptoms. Certain studies have proposed that controlling mast cell release may help with IBS and IBD symptoms. Other research has shown that ingestion of high-histamine foods for individuals with IBS and histamine intolerance or MCAS may make symptoms worse, so removing these foods can help reduce GI symptoms.

Preliminary research has shown that probiotics may reduce GI inflammation, allergy symptoms, and allergenic symptoms such as eczema and atopic dermatitis. Bacteria that help break down histamine in the gut include *Bifidobacterium infantis* and *Lactobacillus plantarum*. Choosing the right probiotic supplement that contains those strains may alter histamine production in your body to your benefit.

If you have IBS, also consider layering a low-FODMAP diet onto this low-histamine, anti-inflammatory diet. The acronym stands for fermentable oligosaccharides, disaccharides, monosaccharides, and polyols, which refer to carbohydrates fermented in your gut by your microbiome. Reducing FODMAP foods for a short period of time and then reintroducing them also can help. In a nutshell, avoid asparagus, beans, beets, broccoli, Brussels sprouts, cabbage, garlic, gluten, lactose, and

onions. You also may want to avoid apples, cherries, honey, mangos, peaches, pears, and plums, which contain large amounts of fermentable sugars. The rest of the low-histamine, anti-inflammatory diet will exclude the rest of the high-FODMAP foods. Milk alternatives include rice milk, oat milk, coconut milk, and Lactaid. Better cheese options include Mascarpone and cream cheese, which have low levels of lactose and histamine. Choose easier-to-digest veggies and consume them cooked rather than raw. These veggies include bok choy, carrots, cucumbers, green beans, lettuce, potatoes, red bell peppers, sweet potatoes, winter squash, and zucchini.

RHEUMATOID ARTHRITIS

Increased number or activity of mast cells has been associated with rheumatoid arthritis, which may increase pain by releasing inflammatory cytokines and histamine. Research has implicated the presence of cytokines such as IL-1, IL-8, and TNF in rheumatoid arthritis and related pain. They also have found increased levels of histamine in the diseased synovium, joint fluid, and inflamed joints of those suffering from RA.

Case control studies have indicated that lifelong consumption of fish, olive oil, and cooked vegetables may have protective effects against the development of RA. Research shows .that a diet high in olive oil and omega-3 fatty acids from fish but low in dairy, gluten, red meat, citrus, tomatoes, and processed foods—essentially an anti-inflammatory Mediterranean diet—improved symptoms in RA patients. A randomized control study by researchers at the Kalmar County Hospital in Sweden, assigned one group of people with RA to follow the Mediterranean diet and another similar size group to consume a normal, nonrestricted diet. The group that followed the Mediterranean diet for three months had a decrease in inflammation and symptoms and increased their physical activity.

A double-blind placebo study by the Albany College of Medicine found that supplementation of fish oil (EPA and DHA) reduced the amount of NSAID-ibuprofen drugs needed to mitigate RA-related pain. Another study by researchers at the National Research Center of Cairo, Egypt, reviewed the activity of bioactive compounds, including *Bifidobacterium bifidum* (probiotic), black cumin (*Nigella sativa*), broccoli, carotenoids (present in carrots), coriander, phytosterols (found in beans), polyunsaturated fats (as in fish and fish oil), rosemary, and sweet potatoes. The consumption of these foods resulted in decreases in inflammatory biomarkers in patients with RA. All of these foods appear in this book for their anti-inflammatory properties.

THE ANTI-INFLAMMATORY CONNECTION

Almost all of the conditions discussed are related to or affected by inflammation, which goes hand in hand with histamine intolerance because overactive mast cells that pump out excess histamine also release inflammatory cytokines, which can cause damage. In the short term, inflammation can help us—such as when our immune system activates to heal a wound—but excessive inflammation over the long term can lead to chronic problems.

As we've seen, many studies indicate that a low-histamine, anti-inflammatory diet can help reduce the symptoms of histamine intolerance, mast cell activation syndrome, asthma, eczema, IC, IBS, IBD, and rheumatoid arthritis. Researchers from the University Clinic of Respiratory and Allergic Diseases Golnik Slovenia found that patients with higher histamine-intolerance symptoms had lower DAO enzyme levels. After following a low-histamine diet for 6 to 12 months, their DAO levels increased. If you don't have enough DAO enzyme, your symptoms will continue to increase in severity. Medical research indicates that the most effective ongoing therapy for histamine intolerance is the limitation of histamine-rich foods.

Diet can increase inflammation in the body or decrease it. The typical Western diet contains excess amounts of processed sugars, refined flours, refined foods, saturated fats, and vegetable oils (high levels of omega-6 fatty acids). These foods, which increase inflammation, include lots of traditional snacks and desserts—crackers, cookies, baked goods—fried foods, and conventional meats. Many of these foods have a higher content of omega-6 fatty acids, which increase arachidonic acid in the body, which in turn increases the release of inflammatory cytokines that increase chronic inflammation. Both omega-6 and omega-3 fatty acids are essential foods, meaning that we need to eat them in our diet, but most people consume too much omega-6. It's imperative to decrease overall intake of omega-6 and increase consumption of omega-3s while balancing insulin levels (affected by eating too much sugar or processed carbs).

The anti-inflammatory food superstars are red fruits and vegetables, orange vegetables, dark green vegetables, purple vegetables and fruits, omega-3 fatty acids from chia seeds, fish, and olive oil, and whole grains. The rich content of vitamins and phytochemicals that they contain provides anti-inflammatory and antioxidant benefits. Eating foods rich in omega-3 fatty acids—chia seeds, omega-3 enriched eggs, and salmon—can reduce inflammation. Using anti-inflammatory herbs and spices such as basil, dill, rosemary, and thyme are great ways to decrease inflammation as well. Olive oil is anti-inflammatory, as is coconut oil, so both make for better choices than butter or vegetable oil when cooking.

Plant-based foods containing polyphenols are among the most effective at inhibiting inflammation. Polyphenols are plant compounds that consist of four groups: flavonoids, lignans, stilbenes, and phenolic acids. Epidemiological studies have found that people who consume foods rich in these polyphenols have a lower incidence of chronic inflammatory diseases. The polyphenols may block cyclooxygenase (COX1 and COX2) and lipoxygenase (LOX), both inflammatory enzymes. Flavonols including quercetin, myricetin, morin, and kaempferol can inhibit LOX pathways. Curcumin (from turmeric) also blocks the activity of the human LOX enzyme

system. When activated, NF-kB—a protein complex that carries genetic material through the body and controls cell survival—increases inflammation and can grow and spread cancer cells. It also can increase allergies, arthritis, asthma, atherosclerosis, and diabetes. Quercetin, found in apples, onions, radicchio, and watercress, suppresses both NF-kB and TNF-alpha, another pro-inflammatory protein. Resveratrol, a compound found in red grapes and wine, also inhibits NF-kB. Purple cabbage and other cruciferous vegetables such as broccoli, Brussels sprouts, and kale contain indole-3-carbinol, another substance that inhibits NF-kB. Eating plenty of apples, onions, red grapes, and watercress and drinking dark grape juice will provide many of these flavonoids. Adding olive oil and nuts to your diet will help reduce inflammation and the risk of chronic inflammatory disease, including cardiovascular disease.

What you eat clearly makes a difference in your overall health and well-being. Eating good-for-you foods should account for 80 percent of your diet. The other 20 percent of the time, you can have a few treats. A low-histamine diet can feel restrictive, but let's not be purists. Food should be wholesome, sure, but it also should feed your soul, which can mean some fun foods with, yes, even a little sugar from time to time!

Contradictions!

Foods & Supplements

By reducing the amount of histamine in your body, you can reduce the amount of inflammation in your cells. Canned fish, cheese, cured pork and sausages, fermented foods, fish sauces, red wine, and sauerkraut all contain elevated levels of histamine. For those who can't process excess histamine, a diet of fresh foods, one that avoids aged or fermented foods, is imperative for maintaining optimal health and well-being. Let's take a closer look at what you should be eating regularly.

FOODS

These foods are great for managing inflammation and histamine-related conditions and reducing inflammatory symptoms. Many of them can stabilize mast cells in the body—and they're delicious!

BASIL

Research has shown that the herb we love in so many dishes reduces cytokine release. Basil also contains rosmarinic acid, a mast cell stabilizer and a potent antioxidant. Try it in some White Bean & Basil Dip (page 85) or White Bean & Basil Cakes (page 120).

BLACK CUMIN (*Nigella sativa*)

Research shows that, when consumed daily, *Nigella sativa* reduces the symptoms of allergic diseases (rhinitis, bronchial asthma, atopic eczema). Study participants reported fewer allergy symptoms when using the seeds or oil. Experimental studies indicate that it blocks histamine release from mast cells. It also protects the gastric mucosal layer, which is especially important for those experiencing GI upset or those with IBS or IBD. You can cook with the seeds or the oil pressed from them. Sprinkle it on your next Carrot, Lentil & Kale Salad (page 95).

BLACK RICE

Forbidden or black rice reduces production of the TNF-alpha and IL-1beta cytokines. It's also rich in anthocyanin, an antioxidant that makes the cooked rice look purple. It cooks up just like long-grain rice and has a nuttier taste that works nicely in Coconut Forbidden Rice Pudding (page 61) or Sesame Chicken (page 194).

COCONUT OIL

Preliminary research has found that the anti-inflammatory properties of coconut oil may reduce the symptoms of arthritis. It's also super easy to cook with! Use it in a batch of Coconut Lemon Bars (page 215) or a Fruit Tart with Mascarpone Cream (page 218). You also can use it topically as a natural moisturizer.

GARLIC

This member of the amaryllis family is a powerhouse of taste, a superfood, and a great anti-inflammatory agent because it reduces the release of inflammatory cytokines from cells. (It's high in FODMAP, though. If you have IBS or IBD, cook with whole cloves that you can remove at the end to avoid aggravating your symptoms.) Whip up a batch of garlic oil to make Garlic Flatbread (page 104).

GINGER

This versatile root reduces the biochemical pathways activated in chronic inflammation. Ginger has anti-allergic potential by stabilizing mast cells. It decreases COX-1 and COX-2 pathways and suppresses leukotrienes, and it also reduces Th2-mediated pulmonary inflammation, as in allergic asthma. Mix up some Soft Ginger Granola (page 32) or Sweet Potato Ginger Muffins (page 54) or grate some into your next dish of scrambled eggs.

HOLY BASIL

Not the same as regular basil, holy basil has exceptional health properties. It stabilizes mast cells, diminishes the release of inflammatory mediators, and in experimental studies reduces anaphylaxis. Pour yourself a soothing cup of holy basil tea the next time you have a helping of Vegetable Coconut Curry (page 168).

OLIVE OIL

An antioxidant and antimicrobial agent, olive oil contains at least 36 phenolic compounds that contribute to its anti-inflammatory value. Consuming olive oil shows promise for reducing the risk of chronic inflammatory diseases. The key, though, is not to overheat the oil, which can oxidize its good fats. Cook no hotter than to medium on the stovetop or 350°F in the oven to preserve the maximum benefits. When choosing olive oil, use the greenest option or first cold press to ensure the highest content of phenolic compounds. The more that producers refine it, as they do with extra-light olive oil, the fewer of these helpful compounds it will contain. But extra-light olive oil is still rich in unsaturated fats and tastes light, so it's great for baking. Use it to make a batch of Purple Sweet Potato Donuts (page 48) or Carrot Apple Cupcakes (page 210).

ONION

This cousin to garlic has a powerful combination of therapeutic components. Onions contain quercetin, thiosulphinate, and other volatile sulphur compounds (hence the smell). These compounds give onions their anti-inflammatory properties, which also have been shown to reduce pain in some animal studies. Onions may prove troublesome for those with IBS symptoms, however. If that's the case for you, cook them thoroughly and try adding them in small amounts to your diet—or use milder scallion greens or chives, which those with IBS symptoms usually can tolerate better. Onions taste delicious on Lettuce-Wrapped Burgers (page 167) or in a Caramelized Onion & Arugula Pizza (page 191).

OREGANO

This quintessentially Italian-American herb contains rosmarinic acid, a mast cell stabilizer that reduces inflammation. Oregano also reduces cytokine release. It's super easy to toss some fresh oregano into a salad dressing, and it will add a hearty zing to your next plate of Spaghetti Squash Pasta with Chicken Meatballs and Pomodoro Sauce (page 192) or Fajita Chicken Rice Bowl (page 163).

PARSLEY

So much more than a garnish, parsley is rich in apigenin, a plant flavonoid that reduces inflammation by reducing production of TNF-alpha, IL-8, IL-6, and COX-2. Sprinkle some on your next salad or add some to a fruit smoothie— it won't make it taste herbaceous, promise! If you want to use it more traditionally, it will go great in your next batch of Garlic Croutons (page 229) or Superfood Stew (page 119).

PEA SHOOTS AND PEA SPROUTS

These are one of the few foods that naturally contain DAO, one of the primary enzymes that break down histamine in the body. Experimental research has shown that DAO from pea shoots may reduce asthma-like allergic reactions and inflammation. Add them to a salad or make Roasted Asparagus with Fried Eggs and Pea Shoots (page 92).

PEPPERMINT

This popular hybrid of watermint and spearmint has a rich flavonoid content. Experimental studies have found that the flavonoid isorhoifolin especially helps reduce histamine release, allergy-related sneezing, and other nasal symptoms when participants consumed peppermint. Peppermint oil has anti-inflammatory, antibacterial, and antifungal properties, and oral intake of enteric-coated peppermint oil effectively reduces IBS symptoms. In a randomized placebo-controlled trial by Robarts Research Institute, two weeks of peppermint oil supplementation showed global improvement in IBS symptoms and improved abdominal pain. Now you have another reason to enjoy a warming cup of peppermint tea or peppermint-infused water! Also try adding some to the Coconut Lemon Bars (page 215).

ROSEMARY

This Mediterranean herb that signifies remembrance contains rosmarinic acid, which decreases inflammatory cytokine release, reduces histamine release from mast cells, and diminishes allergy symptoms that affect the nose, eyes, and skin. It smells heavenly, tastes great in Rosemary Sea Salt Brussels Sprouts (page 136) and Mushroom Rosemary Chicken (page 164), and naturally reduces heterocyclic amine formation—the carcinogens that grilling meat creates.

STINGING NETTLE

Don't let the name scare you! This delicious anti-inflammatory herb may help decrease allergy symptoms. Nettles inhibit mast cell release of histamine, block inflammatory mediators such as cytokines, and may decrease arthritis pain. Looks like it's time to brew up a pot of nettle tea. Try it out in the Vegan Pesto (page 236).

THYME

Like parsley, thyme contains apigenin, a plant flavonoid that reduces cytokine release from mast cells and helps decrease inflammation in the body. In animal studies, thyme acted as an antioxidant and reduced the occurrence of asthma. It also contains thymol, a natural antibiotic and antifungal. You can add it to pretty much anything, including chicken dishes, salad dressings, soups, or stews. Definitely try it in a plate of Maple Thyme Carrots (page 134) or Thyme Garlic Fries (page 145).

TURMERIC

Curcumin is the active anti-inflammatory compound in turmeric that, in experimental studies, reduced inflammation and may inhibit the release of histamine from mast cells. Curcumin reduces allergic rhinitis by suppressing the production of inflammatory cytokines TNF-alpha, IL-1beta, IL-6, and NF-kB. You can add turmeric to many dishes, such as rice, eggs, curries, and vegetables. It works great in the Acorn Squash Soup (page 111) and Vegetable Coconut Curry (page 168).

WATERCRESS

This water-loving plant has lots of flavonoid compounds and megastamines, which significantly reduce the release of histamine. Watercress is also rich in isothiocyanate, vitamin C, and other antioxidants. Its peppery bite makes for a wonderful addition to any salad. Try some in the Butternut Squash & Arugula Salad (page 112).

SUPPLEMENTS

Supplements provide the body with nutrients that food alone can't provide. The following supplements can help with mast cell stabilization, reducing allergies and lessening inflammation, which can help put you on the road to recovery. As you should do before making any dietary change, talk with your doctor before taking any supplements to ensure that no negative interactions will take place with your current medications or other health conditions.

VITAMIN B6

DAO production gets a boost from Vitamin B6. Food sources rich in B6 include bananas, beef, chicken, chickpeas, potatoes, salmon, and turkey. The recommended daily amount is 1.3 mg, which may prove difficult to achieve without supplements.

VITAMIN C

A powerful antioxidant and a mast cell stabilizer, Vitamin C also increases DAO production. For controlling histamine disorders, the suggested dose is 1,000 mg per day.

VITAMIN D

Research has shown that low levels of vitamin D correlate with increased asthma, hives, and other allergy symptoms. Vitamin D decreases the production of cytokines. If you live in extreme northerly or southerly latitudes, you risk developing a vitamin D deficiency in the winter when Earth tilts away from the sun, limiting the UVB rays that reach the surface. Our skin uses those UVB rays to synthesize the vitamin D that our bodies need, so supplementation is crucial in winter. Ask your physician about checking your vitamin D 25-OH levels (the lab name). Most people will need to take 1,000–2,000 IU of vitamin D3 per day, but you might need more if your levels are very low.

LUTEOLIN

This flavonoid shows strong promise as a mast cell stabilizer and reduces the release of cytokines. Rich sources of luteolin include celery, green bell peppers, oregano, parsley, peppermint, pumpkins, radicchio, rosemary, and thyme. Specific supplements contain luteolin if you can't get enough through dietary sources.

MAGNESIUM

Commonly found in black beans, pumpkin seeds, and Swiss chard, magnesium naturally boosts DAO production. The suggested daily dose for magnesium supplementation is 100–300 mg if you don't eat these foods regularly. The recipes in this book use lots of these foods, so they contain plenty of magnesium.

OMEGA-3 FATTY ACIDS

These compounds reduce cytokine release, which causes allergenic responses and inflammation. A diet rich in chia seeds, enriched eggs, fish, and flax oil can increase your levels of omega-3 fatty acids naturally. These foods often make for a better choice than fish oil supplements for histamine-sensitive individuals.

Aim for 1,000 mg per day by diet or with a flax oil or fish oil supplement, the equivalent of eating a 3½-ounce portion of salmon.

PROBIOTICS

Supplementing with beneficial bacteria such as *Bifidobacterium infantis, Lactobacillis plantarum* may help your body produce less histamine and can help with IBS and IBD symptoms.

QUERCETIN

This flavonoid that stabilizes mast cells, acts as a natural antihistamine, and occurs in many foods—especially apples, asparagus, kale, onions, radicchio, and watercress—but you likely need supplementation to reach a functional level in the body in order to see improved symptoms. Research has shown it to be just as effective, if not more, than cromolyn sodium to decrease the release of histamine and other inflammatory molecules. Quercetin has the advantage in that it works preventatively, whereas you have to take cromolyn with the trigger food or else it loses its effect. Suggested dosing for quercetin is 500 mg per day.

ROSMARINIC ACID

This flavonoid decreases cytokine release, reduces histamine output from mast cells, and can alleviate allergy symptoms of the eyes, nose, and skin. It occurs in basil, mint, rosemary, and sage, which you can add to a variety of foods. You also can take it in supplement form.

The Anti-Inflammatory & Low-Histamine Diet

When your levels of histamine and inflammation rise, you need to give your body time and the biochemical tools it needs to break it down. Foods, supplements, and rest will accomplish that goal. The anti-inflammatory and low-histamine diet acts as an elimination diet, meaning that you remove as many no-go foods as you can manage for at least four weeks. Then, if you want, you can add them back, one at a time, to determine your triggers. The triggers and reintroduction time line for each person vary. Some people will need to avoid certain foods for good, but as your histamine levels fall you may be able to tolerate more of your trigger foods than before undertaking the diet.

Remember, the goal here is to reduce inflammation in your diet, not eliminate histamine from it altogether. Histamine occurs in many foods, including fermented foods, slow-cooked meats, deli meats, aged and smoked meats, and cheeses. Many healthy foods also contain histamine, so it's impossible to avoid—but that's OK. You want to reduce histamine intake to allow your body to heal and to process what you do consume. The more anti-inflammatory foods you eat, the quicker your body can do that. Keep foods as fresh as possible and make as much at home as you can. Freeze leftovers so excess bacteria don't grow on them, which can increase histamine levels.

The lists below compile two of the most highly referenced food lists for the low-histamine diet along with dietetic research. (No two low-histamine diet lists are the same.) This diet doesn't account for any personal food sensitivities or allergies, so if you see something on the list that you know you're sensitive or allergic to, avoid that food.

No Tomatoes!!

FRESH VEGETABLES

- ☐ artichokes
- ☐ asparagus
- ☐ beets
- ☐ bok choy
- ☐ broccoli
- ☐ cabbage
- ☐ carrots
- ☐ cauliflower
- ☐ celery
- ☐ corn
- ☐ cucumbers
- ☐ endive
- ☐ fennel
- ☐ green beans*
- ☐ green peas*
- ☐ kale
- ☐ lettuces
- ☐ napa cabbage
- ☐ onions
- ☐ pea shoots or sprouts
- ☐ squash (acorn, summer, winter, zucchini)
- ☐ sugar snap peas
- ☐ sweet bell peppers
- ☐ sweet potatoes
- ☐ Swiss chard
- ☐ watercress
- ☐ white potatoes

* medium intake

FRESH FRUITS

- ☐ apples
- ☐ apricots
- ☐ blackberries
- ☐ blueberries
- ☐ cherries
- ☐ coconut
- ☐ cranberries
- ☐ grapes
- ☐ mangoes
- ☐ melons (cantaloupe, honeydew, watermelon)
- ☐ peaches
- ☐ pears

GRAINS

- ☐ amaranth
- ☐ arrowroot flour
- ☐ corn (cereal— no malt, organic, non-GMO—chips, flour, starch)
- ☐ garbanzo bean flour
- ☐ masa harina (organic, non-GMO)
- ☐ millet
- ☐ oats
- ☐ potato starch
- ☐ quinoa
- ☐ noodles (gluten-free)
- ☐ rice (black, cakes, cereal, crackers, flour, noodles)
- ☐ tapioca starch

NUTS & SEEDS

- ☐ chia seeds
- ☐ flax seeds
- ☐ macadamia nuts
- ☐ pumpkin seeds
- ☐ sesame seeds
- ☐ sunflower seeds

NOTE If you have tolerance issues, limit seeds and nuts to 1-2 tablespoons per day. You can buy fresh nut butter from many health-food stores. When introducing new foods or reintroducing eliminated foods, tree nuts sometimes can prove hard to tolerate at first.

DAIRY

- ☐ butter
- ☐ cream
- ☐ cream cheese
- ☐ farmer's cheese
- ☐ goat milk
- ☐ mascarpone
- ☐ milk (pasteurized)
- ☐ mozzarella (fresh)
- ☐ ricotta

NOTE Large amounts of dairy can be inflammatory, so we'll use dairy minimally in the diet.

FRESH FISH

- ☐ cod
- ☐ haddock
- ☐ halibut
- ☐ salmon
- ☐ trout

NOTE Fish can have somewhat high histamine levels, but you may be able to tolerate it as you lower your own levels. Fish frozen at sea is processed almost immediately, which lessens the time that bacteria can grow on it. Don't defrost it in the refrigerator overnight or all day. Cook from frozen or defrost in the microwave right before cooking.

FRESH MEAT, EGGS & LEGUMES

- ☐ beef (organic, grass fed), small amount
- ☐ black beans (cooked from dry)
- ☐ chicken
- ☐ chickpeas (cooked from dry)
- ☐ duck
- ☐ eggs (cooked)
- ☐ lentils (cooked from dry)
- ☐ navy beans (cooked from dry)
- ☐ pinto beans (cooked from dry)
- ☐ split peas (cooked from dry)
- ☐ turkey

NOTE Choose organic if you can and make sure that meats are neither injected with broth nor marinated. Select as fresh as possible and not temperature abused. Prepare beans from dried—not canned—and freeze any extras.

BEVERAGES

- ☐ coffee (small intake, except if you have tachycardia)
- ☐ espresso (small intake, except if you have tachycardia)
- ☐ fruit juice (100 percent natural, acceptable fruits)
- ☐ herbal teas (peppermint, rooibos, holy basil, etc.)
- ☐ milk (coconut, cow, nut, oat, rice)
- ☐ water (infused with acceptable fruits)

NOTE When choosing a milk, avoid gum additives.

CONDIMENTS, SPICES & BAKING INGREDIENTS

- ☐ ascorbic acid
- ☐ baking powder
- ☐ baking soda
- ☐ basil
- ☐ black cumin (Nigella sativa)
- ☐ cardamom
- ☐ citric acid
- ☐ coconut oil
- ☐ cream of tartar
- ☐ cumin
- ☐ dill
- ☐ flaxseed oil
- ☐ garlic
- ☐ gelatin
- ☐ ginger
- ☐ holy basil
- ☐ lemon or lime juice*
- ☐ mint
- ☐ olive oil
- ☐ oregano
- ☐ parsley
- ☐ pectin
- ☐ peppermint
- ☐ rosemary
- ☐ sage
- ☐ salt (sea salt)
- ☐ stinging nettle
- ☐ sweet paprika
- ☐ thyme
- ☐ turmeric
- ☐ vanilla extract (alcohol-free if sensitive)

SWEETENERS

- ☐ brown sugar*
- ☐ coconut sugar
- ☐ honey (pasteurized)
- ☐ maple syrup
- ☐ stevia
- ☐ white sugar*

* small intake

WHAT TO AVOID

NOTE Avoid anything with artificial ingredients, colorings, flavorings, or preservatives.

VEGETABLES

- x avocados
- x chile peppers
- x eggplant
- x red beans (kidney)
- x spinach
- x tomatoes

NOTE Avoid any vegetable that's canned, fermented, pickled, or made with a sauce from ingredients to avoid.

FRUITS

- x banana
- x kiwi
- x pineapple
- x raspberries
- x strawberries
- x citrus (except small amounts of lemon or lime juice for cooking)

NOTE Also avoid any overripe or dried fruit.

GRAINS

- x buckwheat
- x rye
- x wheat germ
- x whole-grain wheat flour

NUTS

- x almonds
- x cashews
- x pecans
- x walnuts

DAIRY

- x aged cheeses (blue, Cheddar, Parmesan, processed, etc.)
- x milk (unpasteurized)
- x buttermilk
- x sour cream
- x yogurt

NOTE The older the cheese, the more histamine it contains.

FISH

- x fish (that may have been temperature-abused)
- x canned tuna, any other shelf-stable fish, canned or smoked salmon for example
- x crab
- x lobster
- x shellfish

MEAT & LEGUMES

- x meats (aged, broth-infused, deli, dried, marinated, smoked)
- x ham
- x pork
- x salami
- x sausages
- x soybeans
- x tofu

NOTE Especially avoid these items, which all have very high levels of histamine.

BEVERAGES

- **x** alcohol
- **x** citrus juices
- **x** processed energy or sugar drinks
- **x** teas (black, green)
- **x** tomato juice

CONDIMENTS, SPICES & BAKING INGREDIENTS

- **x** allspice
- **x** anise
- **x** bouillon
- **x** caraway
- **x** chocolate
- **x** cinnamon
- **x** cloves
- **x** cocoa
- **x** marinades (most)
- **x** mustard seed
- **x** nutmeg
- **x** pepper
- **x** red wine vinegar
- **x** soy sauce
- **x** vinegar (balsamic, red wine, white wine)
- **x** walnut oil
- **x** yeast (baker's, extract, nutritional)

SWEETENERS

- **x** artificial sweetners
- **x** corn syrup (high fructose)
- **x** malt extract

Kitchen Hacks

- **Invest in good kitchen gadgets.**
A good blender and food processor will save you loads of time and make you more likely to want to cook. Consider buying a lemon squeezer, grater, garlic press, and any other time-saver that catches your eye.

- **Prep lunches on the weekend.**
Once your freezer is stocked, it will amaze you how quickly you can prepare lunch or dinner.

- **Let the grocery store help.**
Purchase prewashed greens and pre-chopped veggies for when you need something fast.

- **Fresh, fresh, fresh!**
Make sure all of your ingredients are as fresh as possible.

- **Prep your veggies.**
Prep on the weekend or the night before to make weekday meals come together quickly. Broccoli, Brussels sprouts, cabbage, cauliflower, green beans, onions, peppers, and sweet potatoes will hold well for 3 to 4 days. Prep salad ingredients that wilt, such as cucumbers and lettuce, no more than one day ahead.

- **Slow-cook veggies but not meats.**
Slow-cooking meats increases their histamine content, but the same doesn't hold true for vegetables.

- **Love your lentils.**
They're the quickest-cooking bean—done in just 20 minutes! Add them to salads, tacos, rice dishes, or soups.

- **Eat lots of bulbs, herbs, and roots.**
Go for fresh basil, dill, oregano, rosemary, and thyme. Grate on the ginger and turmeric. Protect yourself with garlic and onions. Dried are OK, too. Avoid pie spices (allspice, cinnamon, cloves, nutmeg) that are high in histamine.

- **Use extra-light olive oil for baking.**
It tastes light—not like extra-virgin at all—and provides healthier fats for reducing inflammation than other vegetable oils.

- **Try baking without cow's milk.**
You can make all of the baked goodies in this book with non-dairy milks such as coconut, oat, or rice.

- **Cheat with chia.**
  If you can't eat chicken eggs or duck eggs but still want to bake, use one tablespoon of ground flax or ground chia seeds mixed with three tablespoons of water. Let it sit for one to two minutes, then use it as an egg replacement.

- **Spoon out the coconut sugar.**
  You can use it in equal measure to replace granulated white or brown sugar, and its lower glycemic index spikes your blood sugar less. Maple syrup also has lower glycemic levels and provides additional antioxidants and minerals.

- **Make up large batches.**
  Make up large batches of beans (soak for eight hours, then cook), quinoa, and rice. Freeze them in individual portions so you can avoid the cans and always have a quick base for lunch or dinner.

- **Freeze leftovers.**
  As foods age, bacteria levels and histamine can increase, so don't refrigerate them. Frozen leftover meals ensure that you always have something ready to eat that won't trigger unwanted inflammation.

- **Get into a groove.**
  The low-histamine diet requires some planning, but after a while you'll find a good rhythm for achieving all of your food-prep goals!

Recipe Codes

Different people have different dietary restrictions, so it's impossible for one cookbook to be all things to everybody—but, as much as possible, I've tried to include something for everyone. On the pages that follow, you'll see the following recipe codes. Here's what each of them means.

CROWD PLEASER: Great for parties or lots of different palates

DAIRY FREE: You can swap cow's milk for plant milk in all of the recipes in this book, so these dishes steer clear of butter, cheese, and other dairy products.

FAST: Fewer than 15 minutes from start to finish

GREAT SNACK: Perfect for enjoying between meals.

HIGH PROTEIN: These dishes pack a hearty protein punch.

KID FRIENDLY: Little ones will love these.

LOW CAL: Great for snacking between meals or when you want something light

LOW FODMAP: Reduced microbiome-fermentable carbs

SUPERFOOD: Packed with vitamins, minerals, and other nutrients

VEGAN: Totally plant based

VEGETARIAN: Plant based plus dairy and eggs

At the back of the book, you'll find a table of all the recipes along with these codes so that you can search for exactly the dish you want. As the subtitle of the book indicates, all the recipes that follow are gluten-free. They appear in course order (breakfast to dessert) and proceed by the amount of time needed to make them, from shortest to longest. Now let's get cooking!

BREAKFAST

Quick Oats with Berries, Chia & Maple Syrup

A good breakfast doesn't have to take forever to cook. Oatmeal makes a great, fast standby, and quick-cooking steel-cut oats cook in the microwave in just 3 minutes—the ultimate speedy breakfast! The berries provide anti-inflammatory antioxidants, and the chia seeds add an omega-3 boost.

····· FAST · LOW FODMAP · SUPERFOOD · VEGAN ·····

PREP TIME: 2 minutes · COOK TIME: 3 minutes · TOTAL TIME: 5 minutes

½ cup quick-cooking steel-cut oats

⅔ cup water

1 teaspoon chia seeds

½ cup fresh blueberries or blackberries

2 tablespoons maple syrup

1. In a microwave-safe bowl, add the oats and water.

2. Microwave on high for 3 minutes or according to oatmeal package directions.

3. Top with chia seeds, fresh berries, and maple syrup.

Variation

If the weather's too hot for hot oatmeal, make cold overnight oats with this recipe. Put all the ingredients in a glass dish with a lid, substituting ⅔ cup of milk of choice for the water. Cover the dish and refrigerate overnight. Breakfast is ready when you wake up!

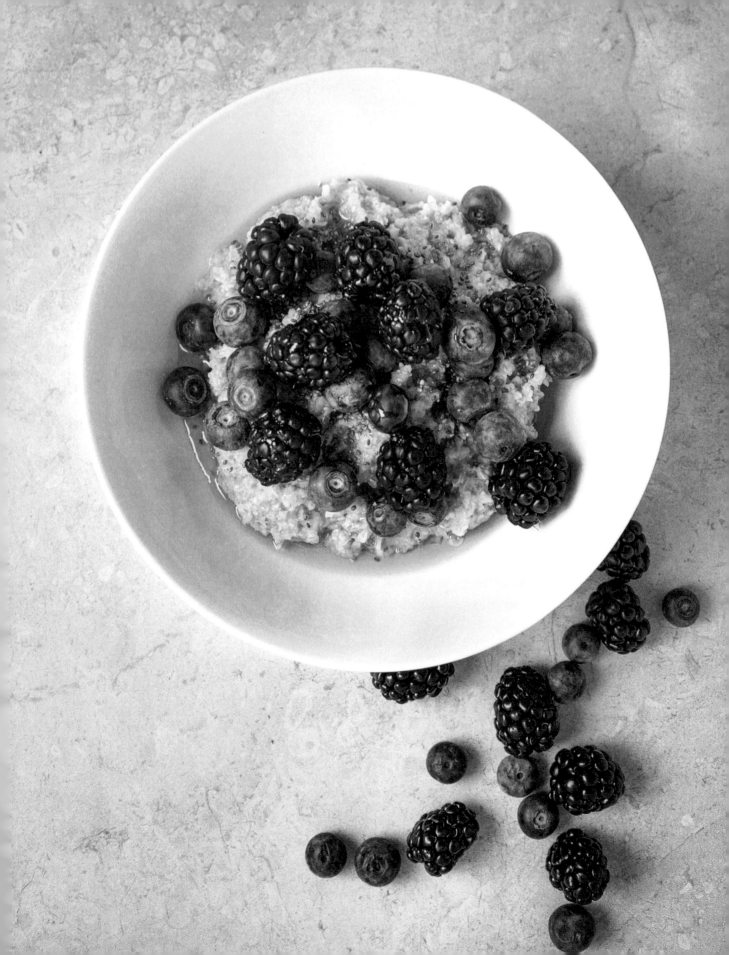

All-Purpose Flour Blend

This flour blend works well in most baked goods. The secret is xanthan gum (or the ground chia seeds), which helps the gluten-free flours stick together. It acts like gluten does in wheat flour, and you can use it in a 1:1 ratio to replace standard all-purpose flour. Mix up a big batch and keep it on hand to use in all kinds of recipes.

····· FAST · LOW FODMAP · VEGAN ·····

PREP TIME: 5 minutes · TOTAL TIME: 5 minutes

1 cup brown rice flour
1 cup white rice flour
3 cups tapioca starch
3 teaspoons xanthan gum

Combine ingredients thoroughly and store in an airtight container or resealable plastic bags for up to 1 month.

Variation

If you're avoiding gums, chia seeds work great as a replacement for xanthan gum. Use it in the following ratio: For 1 teaspoon xantham gum, substitute 1 tablespoon ground chia seeds.

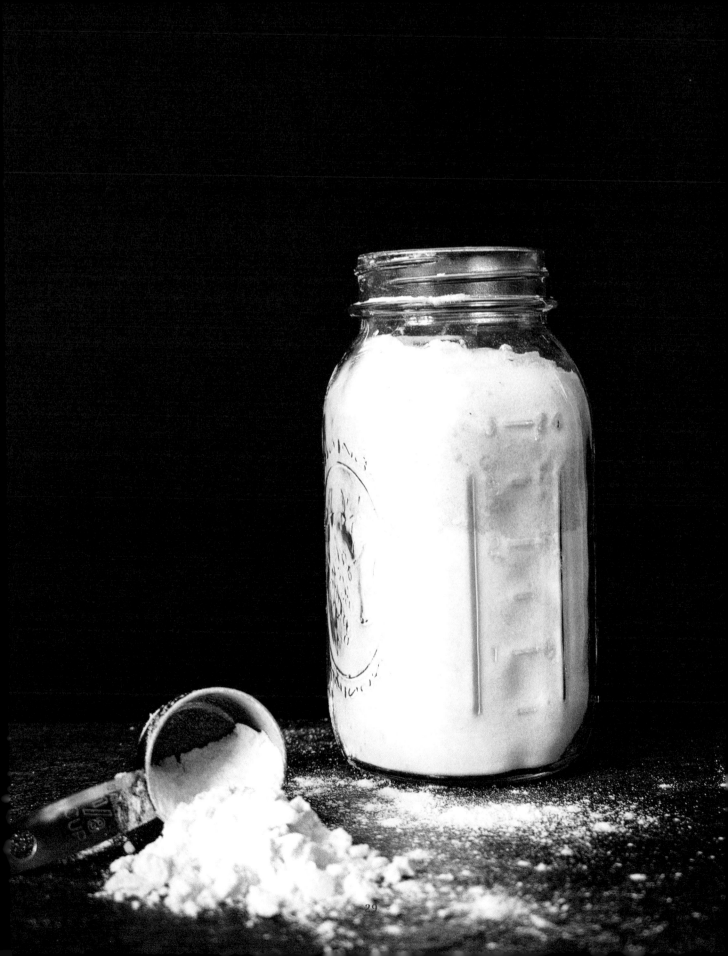

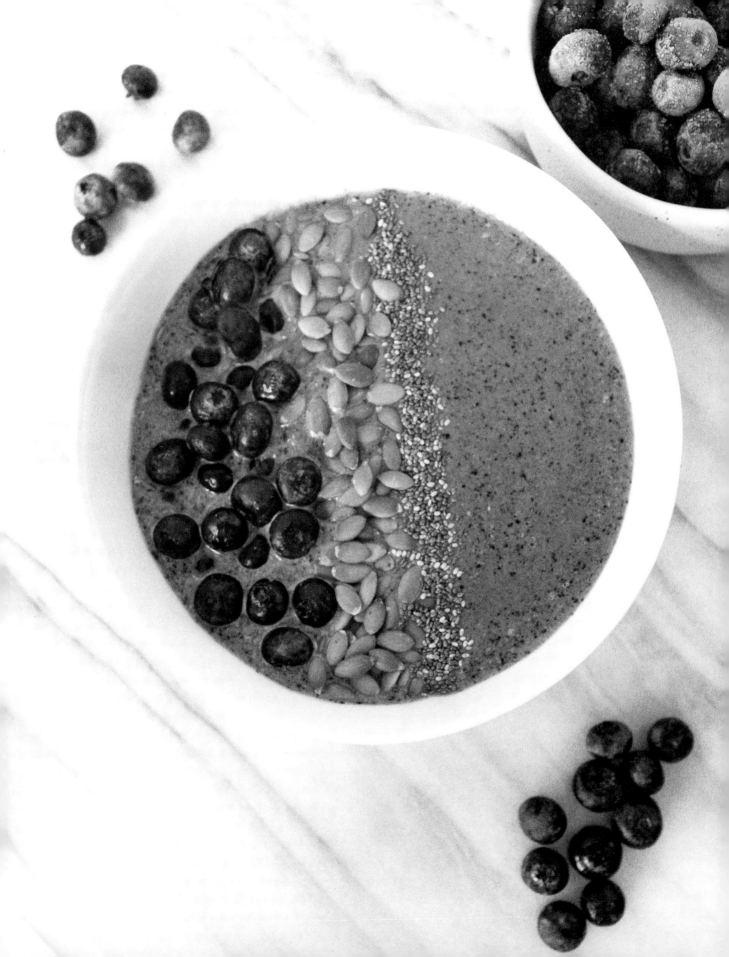

Blueberries & Cream Smoothie Bowl

Smoothies taste delicious, but sometimes they don't feel very filling. To make this one more spoonable, let it sit for about 10 minutes to thicken. Then add your toppings. This is a great five-minute recipe for when you want something quick.

····· FAST · HIGH PROTEIN · LOW FODMAP · SUPERFOOD · VEGAN ·····

PREP TIME: 5 minutes · TOTAL TIME: 5–15 minutes

½ cup frozen blueberries

¾ cup milk of choice

¼ cup rolled oats

2 tablespoons raw pumpkin seeds, plus 1 tablespoon for garnish

1 tablespoon chia seeds, plus 1 tablespoon for garnish

¼ cup fresh blueberries for garnish

1. In a blender, blend all ingredients except garnishes until smooth.

2. If making a smoothie bowl, refrigerate or freeze for 10 minutes to thicken.

3. Top with pumpkin seeds, chia seeds, and fresh blueberries.

> **Note**
>
> *The seeds and oats provide 10 grams of complete plant-based protein, so you don't need to add any protein powder to this dish—although you can if you want some extra oomph in your smoothie / bowl.*

Soft Ginger Granola

This great snack option makes terrific use of ginger, an anti-inflammatory superstar. It tastes like a gingersnap cookie, except it doesn't have all of the baking spices that contain high levels of histamine. So it's good and good for you!

GREAT SNACK · KID FRIENDLY · LOW FODMAP · SUPERFOOD · VEGAN

PREP TIME: 5 minutes · COOK TIME: 20 minutes · TOTAL TIME: 25 minutes

¼ cup extra-light olive oil, plus more for greasing

2 cups rolled oats

½ cup minced ginger

¼ cup raw pumpkin seeds

¼ cup maple syrup

½ teaspoon vanilla extract

¼ teaspoon salt

1. Preheat the oven to 350°F.

2. Grease a 9 x 13-inch glass baking dish with a little extra-light olive oil.

3. In a large mixing bowl, thoroughly combine all of the ingredients. Pour the granola into the prepared baking dish.

4. Bake for 20 minutes, stirring every 5–6 minutes. Don't let the granola become too golden. If you do, it will harden, and you want a nice, easy, soft texture.

5. After 20 minutes or once golden, remove the baking dish from the oven Let the granola cool in the pan on top of the stove or on a wire rack.

Tip

Freeze in airtight single-serving containers or resealable freezer bags for up to 3 months.

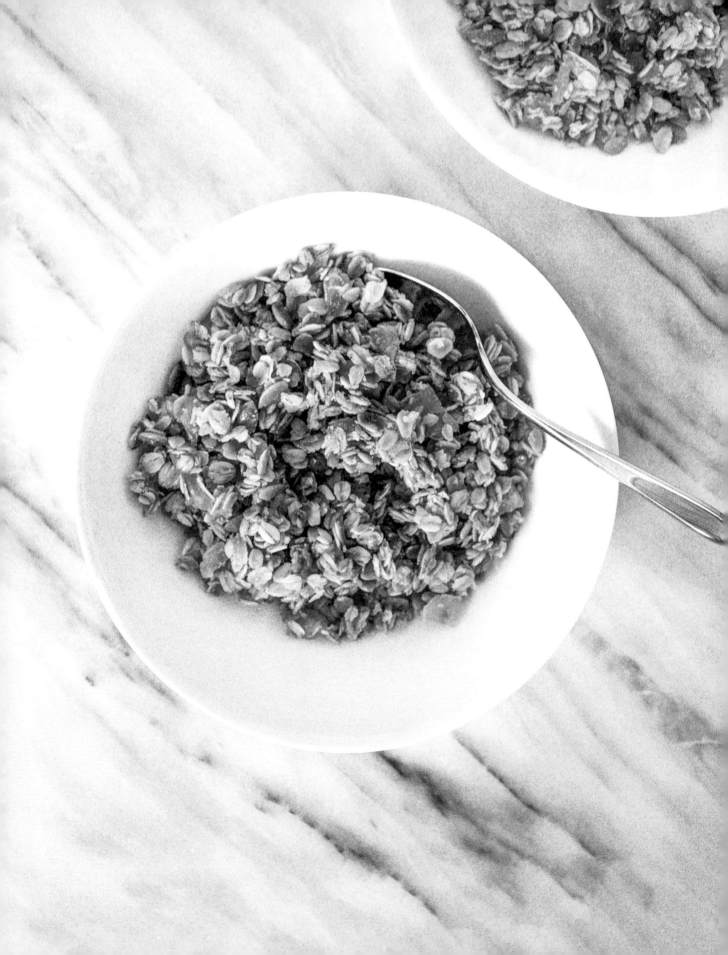

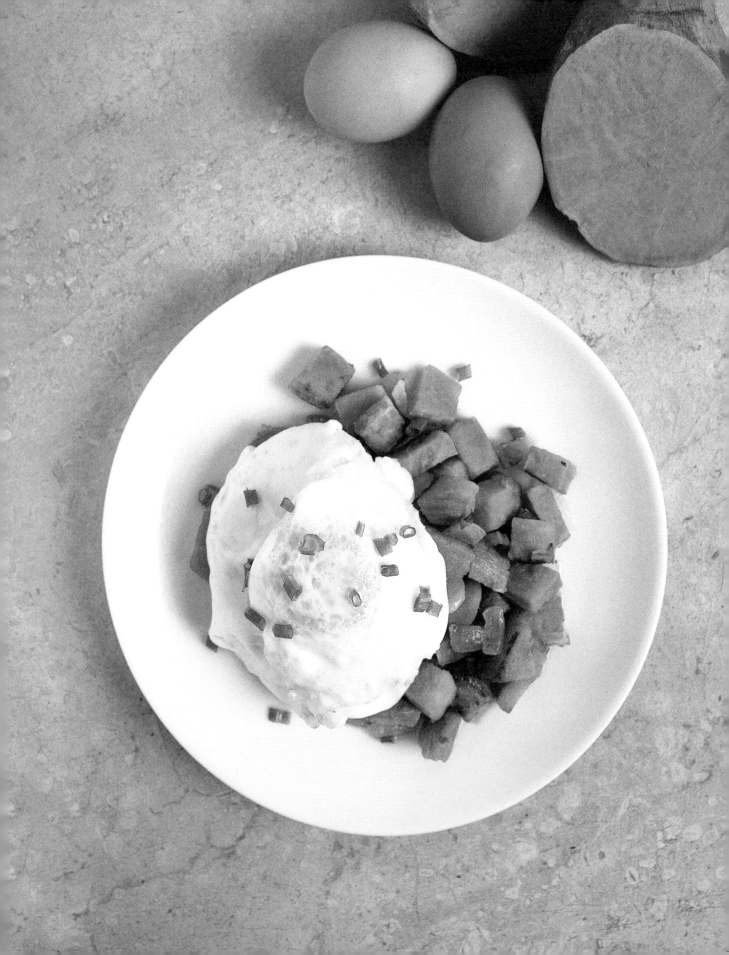

Sweet Potato Hash with Fried Eggs

Adding vegetables to breakfast is a great way to reduce inflammation and boost your recommended veggie intake for the day at the same time. Sweet potatoes and onions add lots of vitamin A and a large breakfast boost of quercetin.

····· CROWD PLEASER · HIGH PROTEIN · SUPERFOOD · VEGETARIAN ·····

PREP TIME: 5 minutes · COOK TIME: 20 minutes · TOTAL TIME: 25 minutes

2 large sweet potatoes, diced

1 red or yellow onion, diced

3 tablespoons olive oil, divided

1 tablespoon butter

salt and pepper

¼ teaspoon smoked paprika

4 eggs

Tip

To make this dish even faster, roast a large pan of diced sweet potatoes and onions coated with olive oil at 400°F for about 20 minutes. Then freeze the mixture in 1-cup portions. You can pull them from the freezer on a busy morning and sauté them in a little more olive oil for about 5 minutes while frying or scrambling a few eggs for a superfast breakfast.

1. Place the diced sweet potatoes in a medium microwave-safe bowl. Add 2 tablespoons of water and cover with a paper towel. Microwave on high for about 4 minutes, until the potatoes are almost tender.

2. In a large skillet, sauté the onions over medium heat in 2 tablespoons of the olive oil and the butter. Cook for about 10 minutes or until tender, stirring occasionally.

3. Add the sweet potatoes to the onions and sauté until the sweet potatoes turn golden, about 5 minutes. Season to taste and add the smoked paprika.

4. In a separate pan, add the remaining 1 tablespoon of olive oil. Crack each of the eggs into the pan, fry them over medium heat to desired doneness, then flip.

5. To serve, layer half of the sweet potato hash on the bottom of the plate and top with 2 fried eggs.

Vegetable Omelet

This veggie-packed, protein-hardy breakfast will keep you feeling full throughout the morning. All of the veggies have tons of antioxidants, which gives you a great excuse for eating them first thing in the morning.

····· HIGH PROTEIN · SUPERFOOD · VEGETARIAN ·····

PREP TIME: 5 minutes · COOK TIME: 20 minutes · TOTAL TIME: 25 minutes

1 tablespoon olive oil
¼ cup chopped kale
¼ cup chopped orange or
   red bell peppers
¼ cup chopped red or yellow
   onions
¼ cup chopped mushrooms
4 eggs
½ cup mozzarella cheese
   (optional)

1. In a medium skillet over medium heat, sauté the vegetables in the olive oil until tender, about 6 minutes, stirring occasionally. Reserve half of the vegetables for the second omelet.

2. Meanwhile, add the eggs into a separate bowl and whip with a fork. Add half of the eggs to the veggies in the pan and cook over medium heat until the bottom sets.

3. Use a spatula to loosen the edges and carefully flip the omelet to cook on the other side. Add cheese to the top if desired and fold the omelet together to melt the cheese.

4. Repeat process to cook the second omelet.

> **Variations**
>
> *If you have a sensitivity to chicken eggs, try duck eggs instead. Omit the cheese for a dairy-free version.*

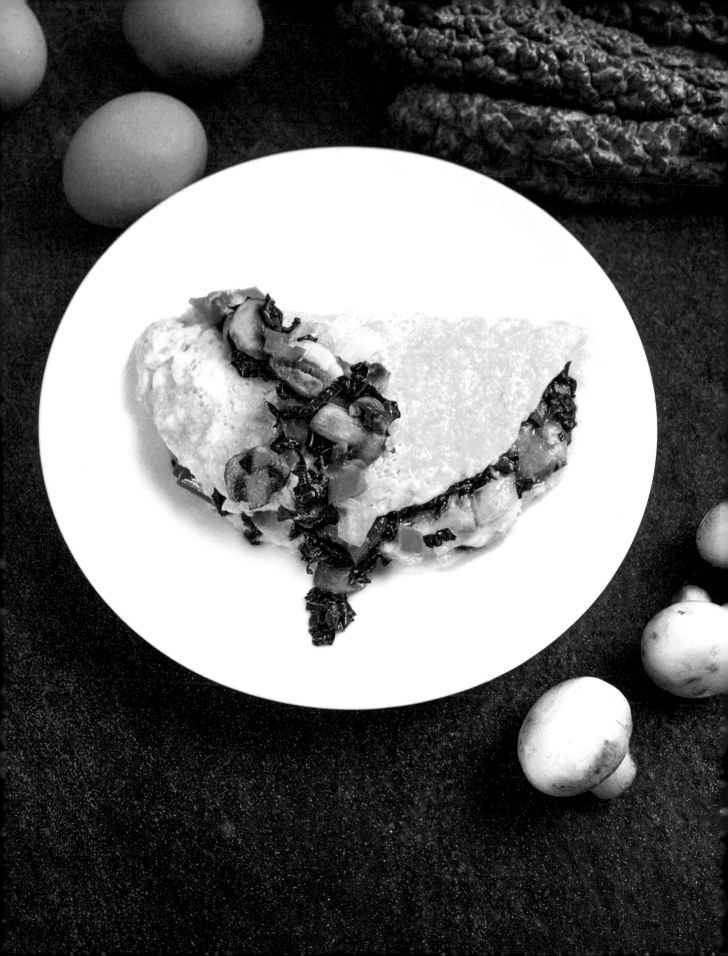

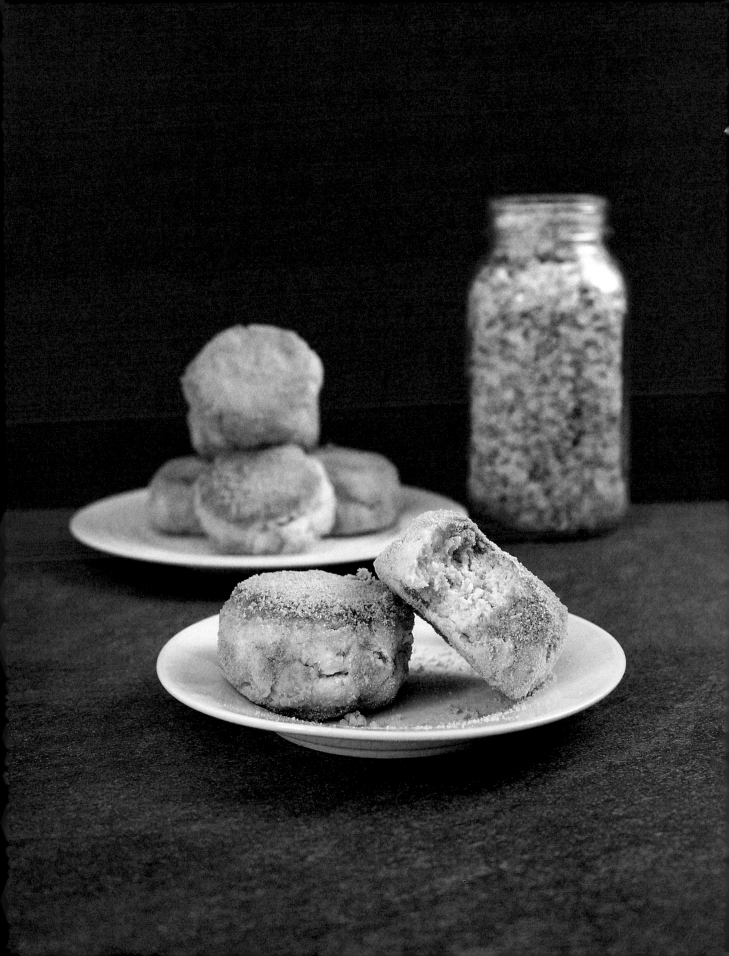

Maple Stovetop Donuts

That's right . . . healthy donuts! These yeast-free treats taste so good that they'll remind you of the real deal. They contain no refined sugar, have just a little crunch on the outside, and the chewy, soft middle has lots of fiber from the oats to keep you full. Coconut oil is naturally anti-inflammatory and naturally sweet, and the maple syrup and maple sugar will satisfy your sweet tooth.

····· CROWD PLEASER · GREAT SNACK · KID FRIENDLY · LOW FODMAP · VEGAN ·····
PREP TIME: 10 minutes · COOK TIME: 15 minutes · TOTAL TIME: 25 minutes

¾ cup quick-cooking steel-cut oats

1 cup milk of choice

¼ cup powdered maple sugar for coating

1¼ cups All-Purpose Flour Blend (page 28)

1 teaspoon baking powder

1 tablespoon maple syrup

2 tablespoons coconut oil, melted

1 pinch salt

¼ cup coconut oil for frying

1. In a medium bowl, combine the oats and the milk. Let sit for 5 minutes so the oats soften.

2. In a separate bowl, add the maple sugar, then set out a large plate lined with paper towels.

3. To the bowl of oats and milk, add the All-Purpose Flour Blend, baking powder, maple syrup, melted coconut oil, and salt and combine well.

4. In a medium skillet, bring the frying oil to medium heat. Add 4 large spoonfuls of dough to the skillet at a time. Using a spatula, shape the batter into even circles. Cover with the lid to increase the rise. Let cook for 3–4 minutes.

5. When the donuts have turned golden brown on the bottom, flip them. Cook on the other side for 3–4 minutes or until golden brown. When the top of the donut feels firm when pressed with your finger, the inside has finished cooking.

6. Remove the donuts from the skillet and toss them in the maple sugar. Repeat with the rest of the dough.

7. Let the donuts rest on the paper-lined plate for 5 minutes until cooled.

Tip

These donuts freeze well for a quick breakfast, snack, or treat.

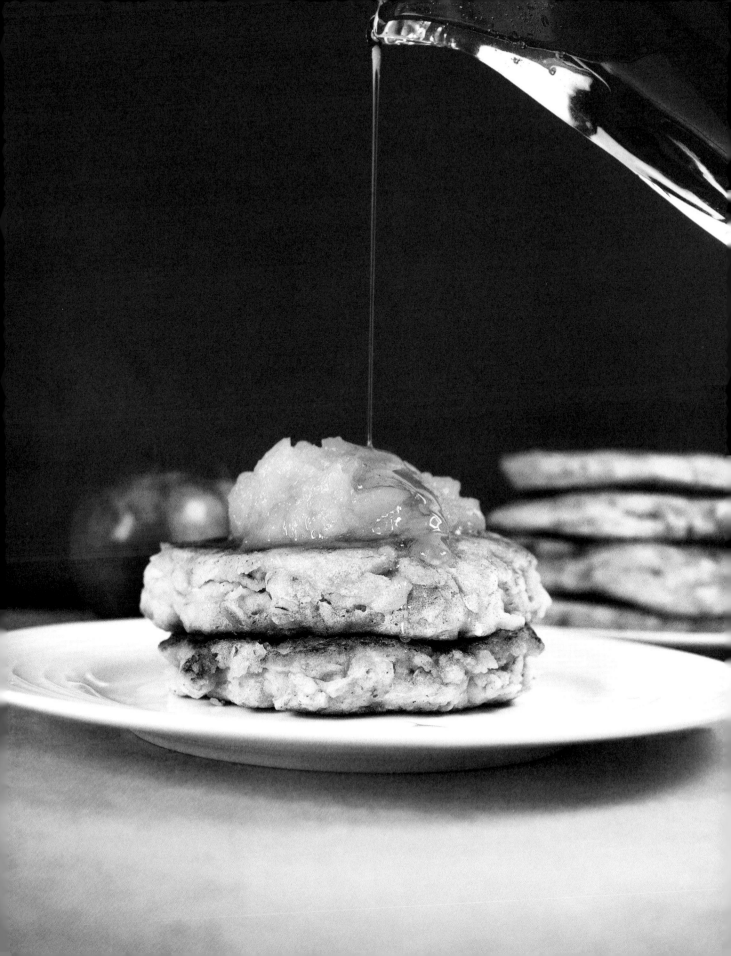

Oat Pancakes with Apple Compote

Pancakes are a great way to sneak some whole grains into your diet, and kids can't resist them. This recipe includes lots of quercetin from the apple in the pancakes and the apples in the topping, helping to decrease inflammation and histamine release.

····· DAIRY FREE · KID FRIENDLY · SUPERFOOD · VEGETARIAN ·····

PREP TIME: 5 minutes · COOK TIME: 25 minutes · TOTAL TIME: 30 minutes

1 cup quick-cook steel-cut or rolled oats

1 cup All-Purpose Flour Blend (page 28)

1 teaspoon vanilla extract

1 teaspoon baking powder

1 tablespoon melted coconut oil, plus 2 tablespoons unmelted (for cooking)

1 egg

1 apple, peeled, cored, and shredded

1 cup milk of choice

APPLE COMPOTE

2 apples, peeled, cored, and diced

2 tablespoons water

1 tablespoon maple syrup, plus more for serving

¼ teaspoon ground cardamom

½ teaspoon vanilla extract

1. Combine the oats, All-Purpose Flour Blend, vanilla extract, baking powder, melted coconut oil, egg, shredded apple, and milk. Mix until the batter just barely forms.

2. In a large frying pan over medium heat, add the 2 tablespoons unmelted coconut oil.

3. Add 4 scoops of batter and cook about 2–3 minutes per side or until golden and cooked through.

4. In a medium pan over medium heat, sauté the apples in the water, maple syrup, and cardamom for about 10 minutes or until the apples are tender.

5. Mash the apples and mix in the vanilla extract at the very end.

6. Top with additional maple syrup if desired.

> **Tip**
>
> *Use a potato masher to mash the apples in no time flat.*

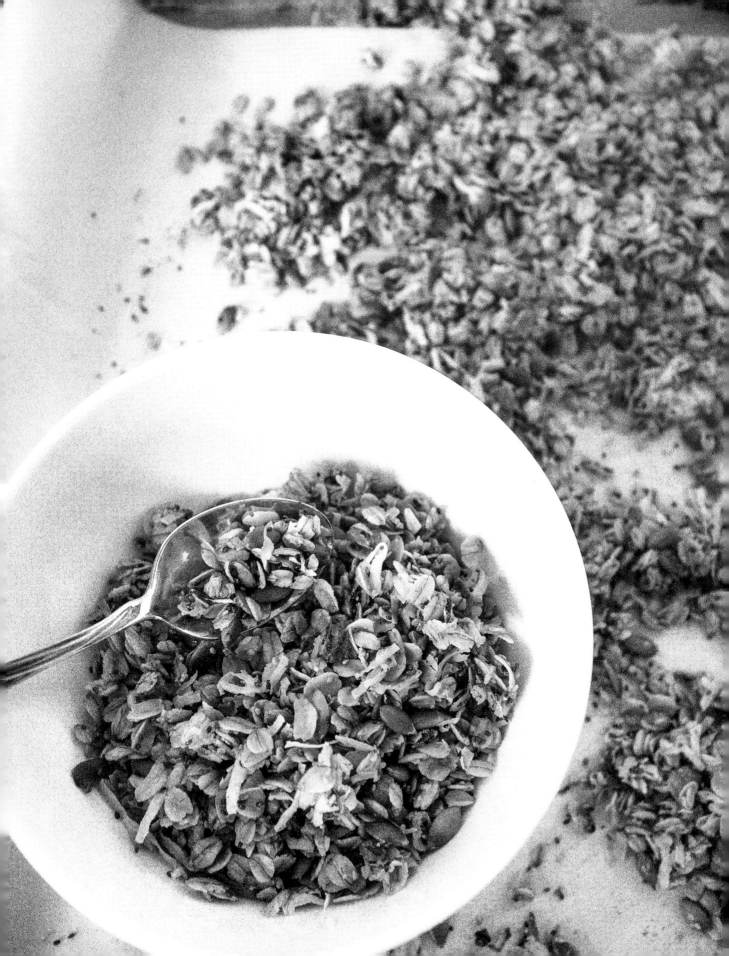

Coconut Crunch Granola

This granola has just the right amount of crunch and flavor. Pumpkin seeds and chia seeds add magnesium, zinc, and anti-inflammatory omega-3 fatty acids. It's also rich in whole grains and good fats and makes a great snack option. It's so easy to make that you won't ever have to buy granola again.

····· GREAT SNACK · SUPERFOOD · VEGAN ·····

PREP TIME: 5 minutes • COOK TIME: 25 minutes • TOTAL TIME: 30 minutes

2 cups rolled oats

½ cup shredded coconut (unsulfured, no preservatives, unsweetened)

¼ cup raw pumpkin seeds

¼ cup maple syrup

¼ cup extra-light olive oil

2 tablespoons chia seeds

1. Preheat the oven to 350°F.

2. Line a baking sheet with parchment paper.

2. In a large mixing bowl, combine all the ingredients.

3. Spread the granola in a single layer on the pan. Bake for 20–25 minutes until golden brown, stirring at about 10 minutes.

4. Once golden, remove the baking dish from the oven. Let the granola cool in the pan on top of the stove or on a wire rack.

Tip

You can store this dish for up to 3 days at room temperature or freeze in airtight single-serving containers or resealable freezer bags for up to 3 months.

Cornmeal Waffle Egg Sandwiches

These delightfully savory breakfast sandwiches are a mash-up of fried eggs and waffles with syrup. Choose omega-3-fortified eggs or organic eggs to boost your omega-3 levels, which can reduce inflammation. Using half olive oil and half butter allows the rich taste of butter to shine in the finished dish but with less saturated fat. The scallions add antioxidants and a nice bright vegetal taste to balance the earthiness of the waffles.

····· CROWD PLEASER · LOW FODMAP · VEGETARIAN ·····

PREP TIME: 5 minutes · COOK TIME: 30 minutes · TOTAL TIME: 35 minutes

¼ cup melted butter

¼ cup extra-light olive oil, plus 1 tablespoon for frying

2 eggs for the batter, plus 12 eggs for frying

½ cup cornmeal

½ cup corn flour

1 cup All-Purpose Flour Blend blend (page 28)

2 tablespoons chopped scallions, plus 1 tablespoon for garnish

2 tablespoons maple syrup

2 teaspoons baking powder

½ teaspoon salt

1½ cups milk of choice

maple syrup for serving (optional)

1. Preheat the waffle iron.

2. In a mixing bowl, combine the butter, oil, 2 eggs, cornmeal, corn flour, All-Purpose Flour Blend, scallions, maple syrup, baking powder, salt, and milk. Mix together until smooth.

3. Prepare the hot waffle iron with olive oil spray and pour roughly a third of the batter onto the iron.

4. In a skillet over medium heat, fry 6 eggs with the remaining tablespoon of olive oil for 90 seconds or to desired doneness. Cook remaining 6 eggs if cooking for a crowd.

5. Place a fried egg each atop a waffle quarter, then top with a second waffle quarter. Drizzle with maple syrup if desired and garnish with scallions.

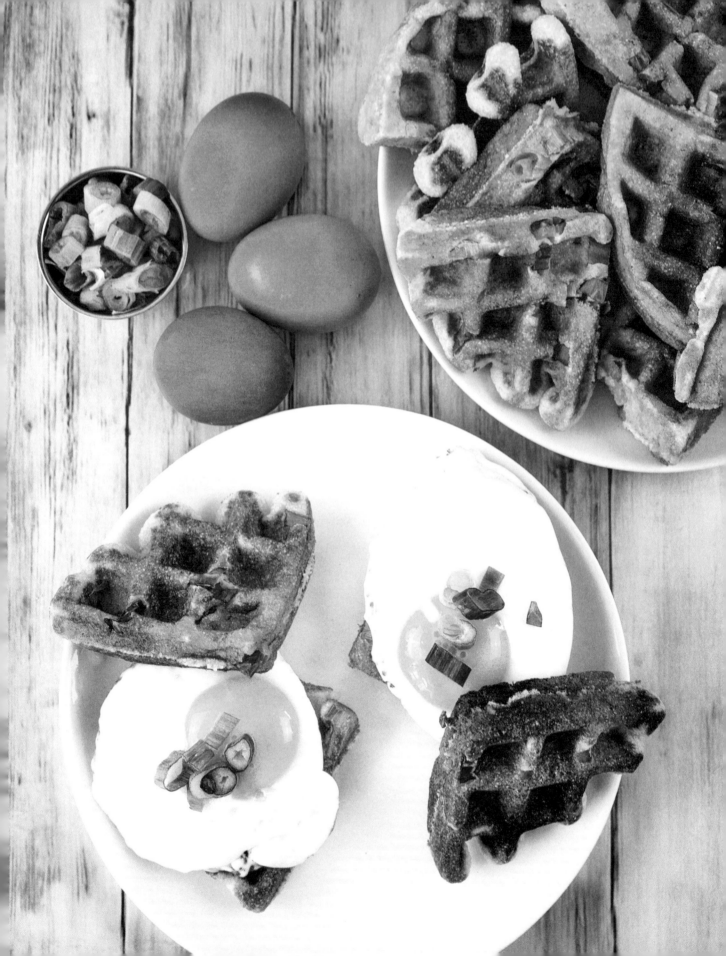

Oatmeal Rolls

Oats are a great way to increase the nutrition of starchy baked goods, and they also help to stabilize your blood-sugar levels. You can freeze these rolls for a quick side to a meal, and they also serve as a sturdy base for all kinds of sandwiches.

····· DAIRY FREE · LOW FODMAP · VEGETARIAN ·····

PREP TIME: 10 minutes • COOK TIME: 25 minutes • TOTAL TIME: 35 minutes

¼ cup extra-light olive oil, plus 1 tablespoon for greasing

½ cup rolled oats, plus ¼ cup for topping

2 cups All-Purpose Flour Blend (page 28)

1 egg

1 tablespoon coconut sugar or maple syrup

1 teaspoon baking powder

1 pinch salt

⅓ cup milk of choice

1. Preheat the oven to 350°F.

2. Lightly grease a small loaf pan with 1 tablespoon olive oil.

3. In a mixing bowl, combine the oats, All-Purpose Flour Blend, egg, olive oil, sugar or syrup, baking powder, and salt.

4. Add the milk, stir to combine, and pour into a loaf pan, filling almost all of the way.

5. Divide the extra oats on top of each roll.

6. Bake for 20–25 minutes until they turn golden brown and a toothpick inserted in the middle of a roll comes out clean.

> **Tip**
>
> *To defrost frozen rolls, microwave for 15–20 seconds.*

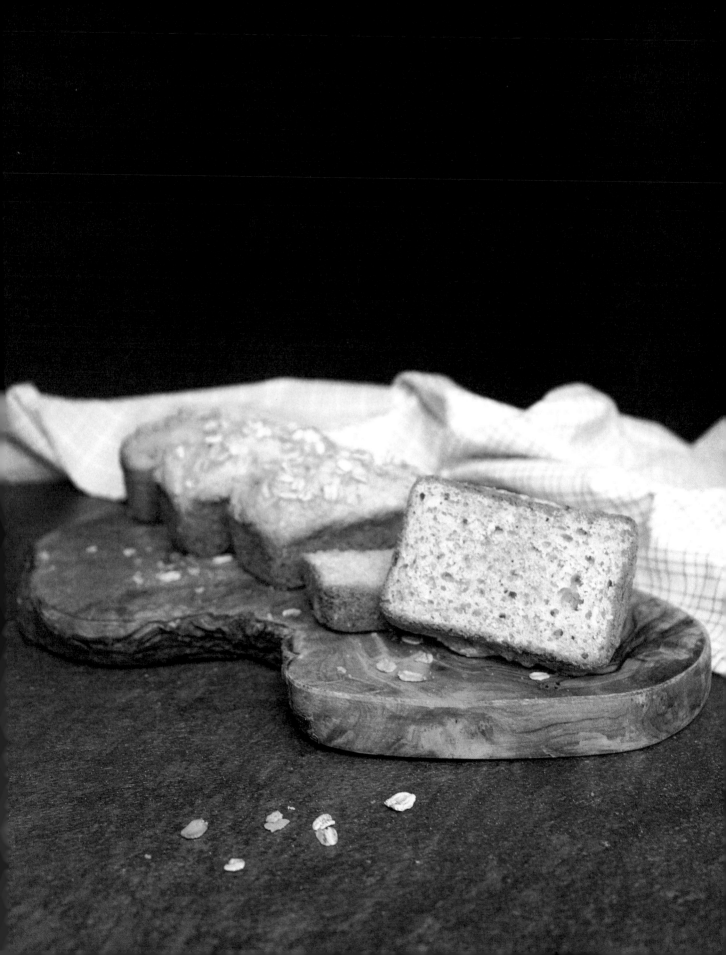

Purple Sweet Potato Donuts

Everyone should eat more purple foods, and this is an easy, delicious way to do that . . . while sneaking more veggies into the mix. The purple pigment in the sweet potato is anthocyanin, a potent antioxidant. The smokiness of the potato enhances and balances the vanilla in this dish, while the oats provide lots of fiber and protein to help you stay full all morning. These donuts aren't fried, so they're healthier than store-bought, but you will need donut pans to bake them.

····· CROWD PLEASER · DAIRY FREE · GREAT SNACK · KID FRIENDLY ·····
SUPERFOOD · VEGETARIAN

PREP TIME: 15 minutes · COOK TIME: 20 minutes · TOTAL TIME: 35 minutes

½ cup extra-light olive oil,
    plus more for greasing
1 medium purple sweet
    potato
½ cup maple syrup
1 teaspoon vanilla extract
⅓ cup milk of choice
2 eggs
1⅓ cups rolled oats
1½ cups All-Purpose Flour
    Blend (page 28)
1 teaspoon baking powder
1 pinch salt

FROSTING (*optional*)

1 (13½) ounce can coconut
    cream (refrigerated for
    24 hours)
1 tablespoon maple syrup

1. Preheat the oven to 350°F.

2. Grease your donut pans with a little olive oil.

3. Poke a few holes into the sweet potato, wrap it in a wet paper towel, and microwave on high for 5 minutes. Allow it to cool for a few minutes, then peel off the skin and discard or save for alternate use.

4. In the bowl of a stand mixer, combine 1 cup cooked sweet potato, olive oil, maple syrup, vanilla extract, milk, and eggs. Mix until well combined.

5. In a food processor, pulse the rolled oats until they grind into 1 cup of oat flour.

6. Add the oat flour, All-Purpose Flour Blend, baking powder, and salt to the sweet potato mixture. Mix again until well combined.

7. Add the batter to the cavities in the donut pan(s) until each is about ¾ full. Bake for 15–20 minutes. They're done when a toothpick inserted in the middle of a donut comes out clean.

8. Let the donuts cool completely in the pan before eating or topping with frosting.

9. If making the frosting, scoop out the solids from the can of chilled coconut cream. Discard or save the remaining coconut water for alternate use.

10. In the bowl of a stand mixer, add the congealed coconut cream and maple syrup. Whip until they combine and become fluffy.

11. Dip the top of each donut in the frosting and chill in the refrigerator for 30 minutes to firm.

Tip

For a quick snack or breakfast option, freeze the donuts in airtight single-serving containers or resealable freezer bags for up to 3 months.

Variation

If you can't find purple sweet potatoes, you can use a regular sweet potato.

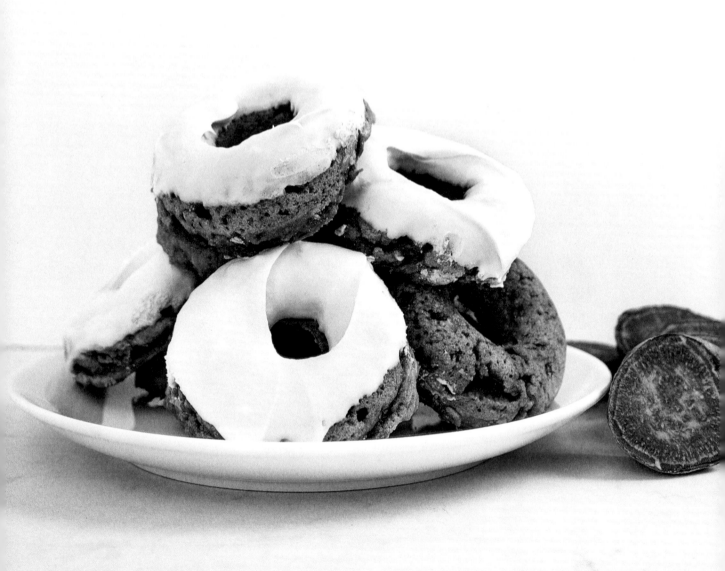

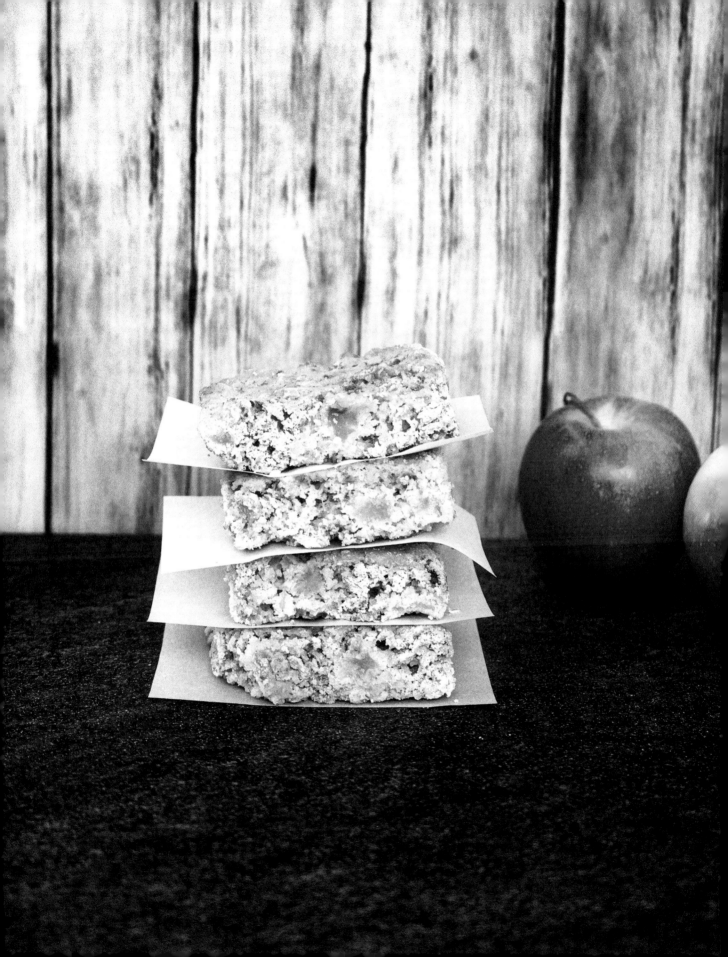

Apple Oatmeal Bars

This breakfast on the go also makes for a great snack. Filled with oats, apples, and pumpkin seeds, these bars will keep you feeling full. Pumpkin seeds add a good amount of magnesium, omega-3 fatty acids, and protein. Apples are rich in quercetin, so an apple a day helps keep the histamine at bay.

····· CROWD PLEASER · DAIRY FREE · GREAT SNACK · KID FRIENDLY ·····
SUPERFOOD · VEGETARIAN

PREP TIME: 5 minutes · COOK TIME: 35 minutes · TOTAL TIME: 40 minutes

½ cup coconut oil, plus more for greasing

½ cup coconut sugar or maple syrup

1 teaspoon vanilla extract

2 eggs

2 red apples, peeled, cored, and diced or grated

3 tablespoons milk of choice

1⅙ cups rolled oat flour, divided

2 cups All-Purpose Flour Blend (page 28)

¼ teaspoon salt

1 teaspoon baking powder

¼ cup pumpkin seeds (see Tip below)

1. Preheat the oven to 375°F.

2. Grease a 9 x 13-inch baking dish with some coconut oil.

3. In the bowl of a stand mixer, combine the rest of the coconut oil and coconut sugar or maple syrup and mix until they combine.

4. Add the vanilla extract, eggs, apples, and milk and mix until they combine.

5. In a food processor, pulse ⅔ cups of rolled oats into ½ cup of oat flour.

6. Add the oat flour, All-Purpose Flour Blend, oats, salt, baking powder, and pumpkin seeds to the apple mixture. Mix until they just combine.

7. Spread the batter into the prepared baking dish and bake for 30–35 minutes, until the topping turns golden brown.

8. Remove the bars from the oven and let cool for 30 minutes or more time, if needed. Cut into bars using a knife.

Tip

If you don't like the texture of seeds in your baked goods, grind the pumpkin seeds into a powder.

Blueberry Corn Muffins

Muffins are incredibly convenient for breakfast or as a snack. Make up a batch, as below, freeze them to keep them fresh, then thaw them as needed by microwaving for 15-20 seconds. Blueberries are one of the easiest ways to add antioxidants to any dish—especially breakfast.

····· DAIRY FREE · GREAT SNACK · KID FRIENDLY · LOW FODMAP ·····
SUPERFOOD · VEGETARIAN

PREP TIME: 10 minutes • COOK TIME: 30 minutes • TOTAL TIME: 40 minutes

1 egg

⅔ cup maple syrup or
    coconut sugar

1¼ cup extra-light olive oil

1 cup cornmeal, organic,
    non-GMO

1½ cups All-Purpose Flour
    Blend (page 28)

1 teaspoon baking powder

1 cup milk of choice

1½ cups blueberries, frozen
    or fresh

1. Preheat oven to 350°F.

2. Line a 12-cup muffin tin with parchment-paper liners.

3. In a large mixing bowl, combine egg, syrup or sugar, olive oil, cornmeal, flour, baking powder, and milk. Stir until mostly combined, then add the blueberries.

4. Pour batter into each lined muffin tin, filling them almost all the way full. Gluten-free muffins don't rise as much as wheat-flour muffins.

5. Bake for 25–30 minutes until the tops turn golden brown and a toothpick inserted in the middle of a muffin comes out clean.

> **Variation**
>
> *This recipe goes nicely with other anti-inflammatory fruits as well. Try making them with mangoes or peaches for summer variety.*

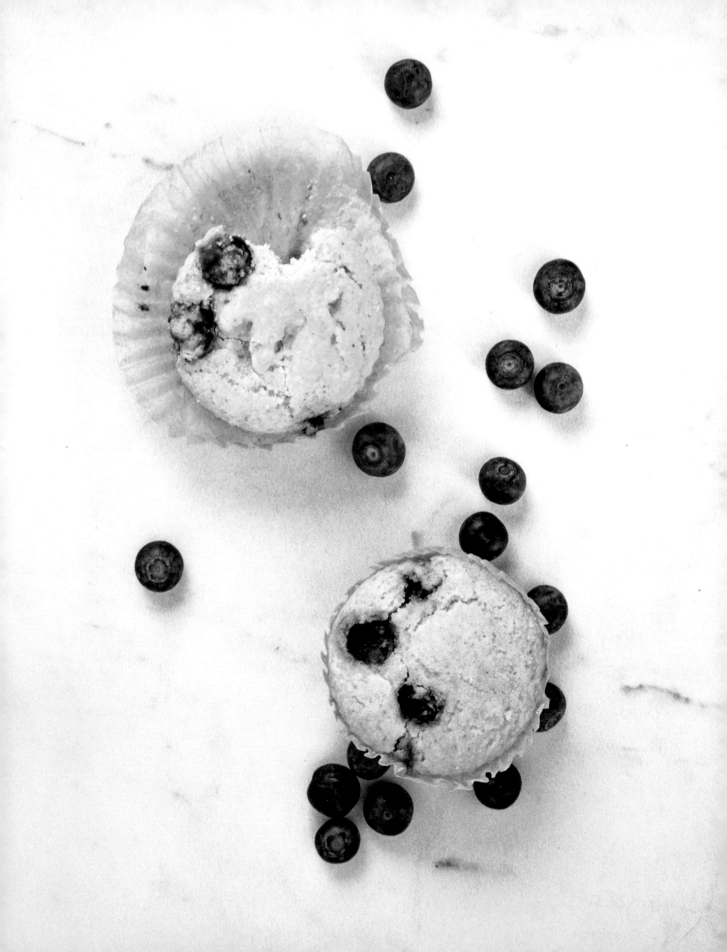

Sweet Potato Ginger Muffins

These antioxidant-packed muffins pair up with the anti-inflammatory goodness of ginger and sweet potatoes, and they're a great way to eat more veggies or sneak them into your kids' diets.

····· DAIRY FREE · GREAT SNACK · LOW FODMAP · SUPERFOOD · VEGETARIAN ·····
PREP TIME: 15 minutes • COOK TIME: 25 minutes • TOTAL TIME: 40 minutes

1 medium sweet potato
½ cup maple syrup
⅓ cup extra-light olive oil, plus more for greasing (optional)
1 egg
1 tablespoon grated fresh ginger
⅔ cup milk of choice
1 teaspoon vanilla extract
1⅓ cups rolled oats
1½ cups All-Purpose Flour Blend (page 28)
1 teaspoon baking powder
¼ teaspoon salt

1. Preheat the oven to 350°F.

2. Grease a 12-cup muffin tin with extra-light olive oil or line it with parchment-paper liners.

3. Poke a few holes in the sweet potato, wrap it in a wet paper towel, and microwave on high for about 5 minutes, until tender.

4. Allow to cool for a few minutes, remove the skin, and discard or save it for alternate use. Mash the flesh.

5. In a medium bowl, combine the sweet potato with the maple syrup, oil, egg, ginger, milk, and vanilla extract and mix well.

6. In a food processor, pulse the rolled oats into 1 cup of oat flour. Add the oat flour, All-Purpose Flour Blend, baking powder, and salt to the sweet potato mixture. Stir gently until the mixture just combines.

7. Fill the muffin tins to the top with batter. Gluten-free muffins don't rise as much as wheat-flour muffins. Bake for 20–25 minutes or until a toothpick inserted in the middle of a muffin comes out clean.

Tip

For a quick breakfast or snack, freeze extra muffins in airtight single-serving containers or resealable freezer bags for up to 3 months.

Variation

Extra-light olive oil is great for baking because it doesn't taste like anything. If you prefer it, coconut oil works nicely in this recipe as well.

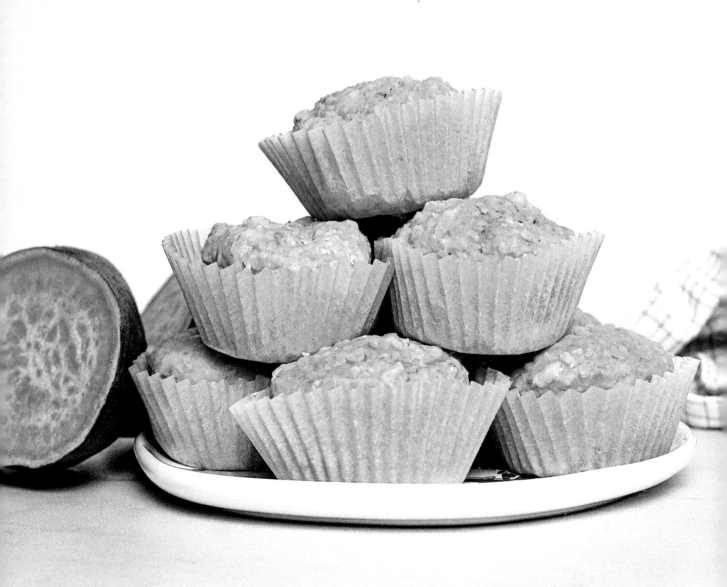

Maple Scones

These delicious treats taste more like dessert than breakfast, but they won't send your blood sugar skyrocketing and then crashing like conventional desserts. The oats and pumpkin seeds add fiber, zinc, magnesium, and protein to what otherwise wouldn't be quite so healthy an option. But hey, a little fun food makes for a balanced diet!

····· CROWD PLEASER · GREAT SNACK · KID FRIENDLY · VEGETARIAN ·····

PREP TIME: 20 minutes • COOK TIME: 20 minutes • TOTAL TIME: 40 minutes

1 cup rolled oats

1¾ cups All-Purpose Flour Blend (page 28)

¼ cup ground pumpkin seeds

1 teaspoon baking powder

9 tablespoons butter

¼ cup maple syrup

1 teaspoon vanilla extract

1 egg

¼ teaspoon salt

¼ cup milk of choice

¼ cup raw sugar

Variation

Butter and scones go together like a horse and carriage, but for a dairy-free version, you can substitute hard coconut oil.

1. Preheat the oven to 375°F.

2. Line a baking sheet with parchment paper.

3. In a food processor, pulse the rolled oats into ¾ cup of oat flour. In a large mixing bowl, combine the oat flour, All-Purpose Flour Blend, ground pumpkin seeds, and baking powder.

4. Using a pastry blender, cut the butter into ¼-inch pieces and combine.

5. Add the maple syrup, vanilla extract, egg, and milk and combine until the dough forms into a ball.

6. Onto a floured board, press the dough out by hand into a 1-inch-thick circle.

7. Cut out 12 scone-shaped triangles from the dough and lay them on the prepared baking sheet. Sprinkle the tops with a little sugar.

8. Bake for 15–20 minutes until the scones turn golden brown on the bottom. They're hard to resist, but let them cool completely on a wire rack, about 5 minutes, before eating.

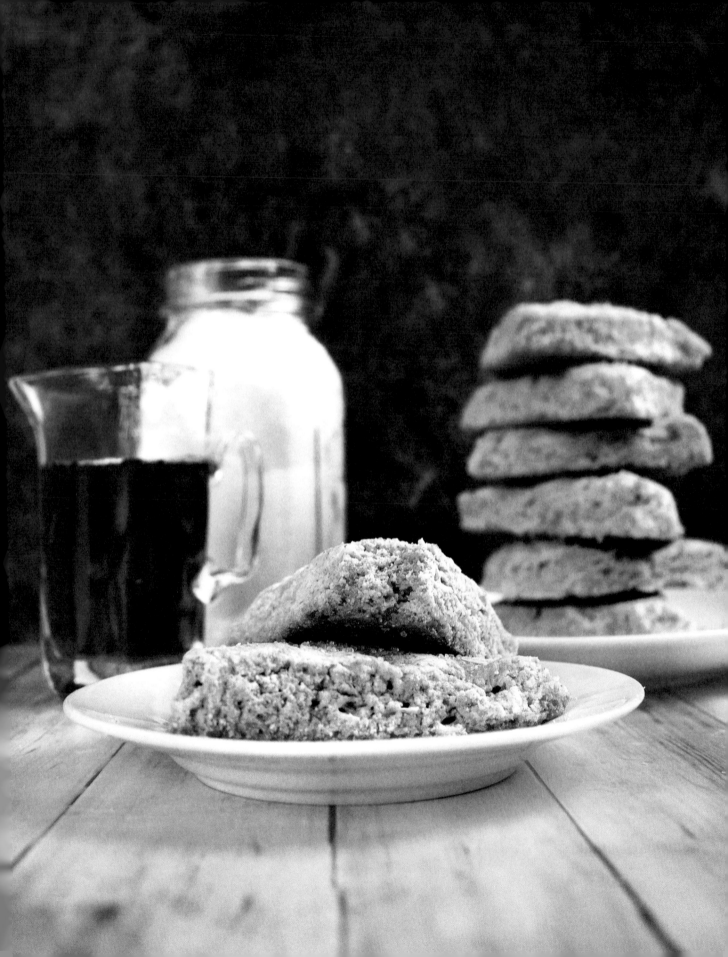

Soft Oatmeal Bread

Everyone needs bread! This cookbook is yeast-free, so this finished dish won't be as sturdy as a yeast bread and resembles a quick bread more in texture. Try making it in a cake pan, as below, and slicing triangles for breakfast or as sandwich bread. Coconut sugar and maple syrup each have a lower glycemic index than regular sugar, and the ground pumpkin seeds increase the zinc, antioxidant, and good-fat content of this bread—even though you can't taste them in there!

····· DAIRY FREE · LOW FODMAP · VEGETARIAN ·····

PREP TIME: 15 minutes • COOK TIME: 30 minutes • TOTAL TIME: 45 minutes

¼ cup extra-light olive oil, plus more for greasing

1⅓ cups rolled oats, plus 2 tablespoons for topping

¼ cup ground pumpkin seeds

1½ cups All-Purpose Flour Blend (page 28)

1 teaspoon baking powder

½ teaspoon salt

¼ cup coconut sugar or maple syrup

1 cup milk of choice

2 eggs

1. Preheat the oven to 375°F. and grease an 8-inch cake pan with extra-light olive oil.

2. In a food processor, pulse the rolled oats into 1 cup of oat flour.

3. In a mixing bowl, combine the oat flour, ground pumpkin seeds, All-Purpose Flour Blend, baking powder, salt, and sugar or syrup and mix together.

4. Add the milk, eggs, and oil and mix until they just combine.

5. Pour the batter into the pan and, with wet hands, pat it down until smooth. Sprinkle the rolled oats on top.

6. Bake for about 30 minutes or until the bread turns golden brown on top and a toothpick inserted in the middle of the bread comes out clean.

7. Let cool on a wire rack and cut into 10 triangular pieces.

> **Tip**
>
> *Freeze any remaining slices in airtight single-serving containers or resealable freezer bags for up to 2 months or turn them into Garlic Croutons (page 229).*

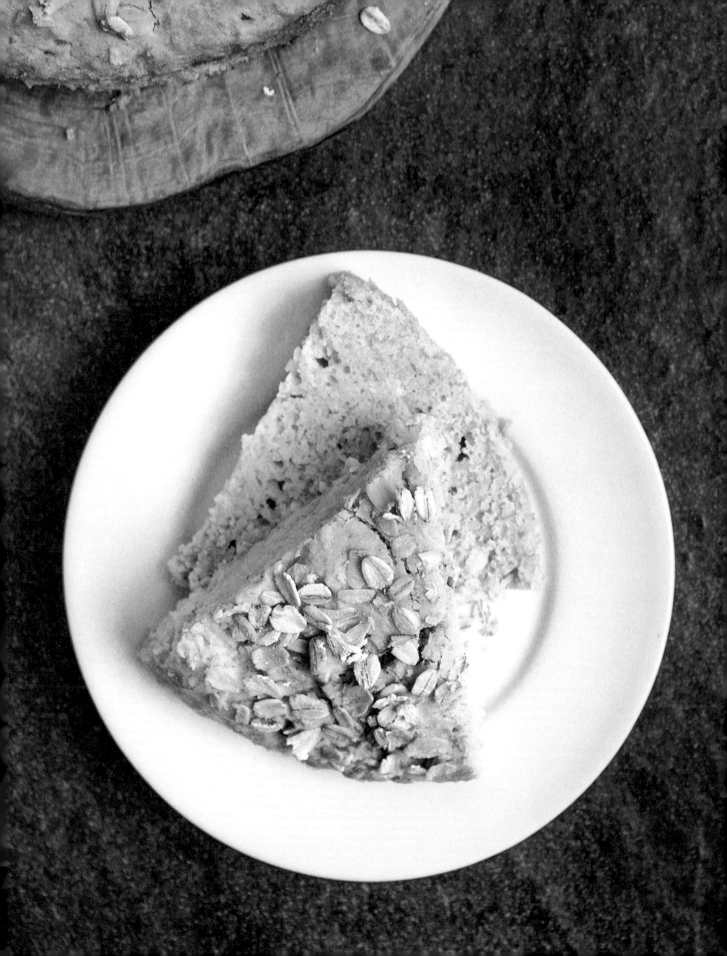

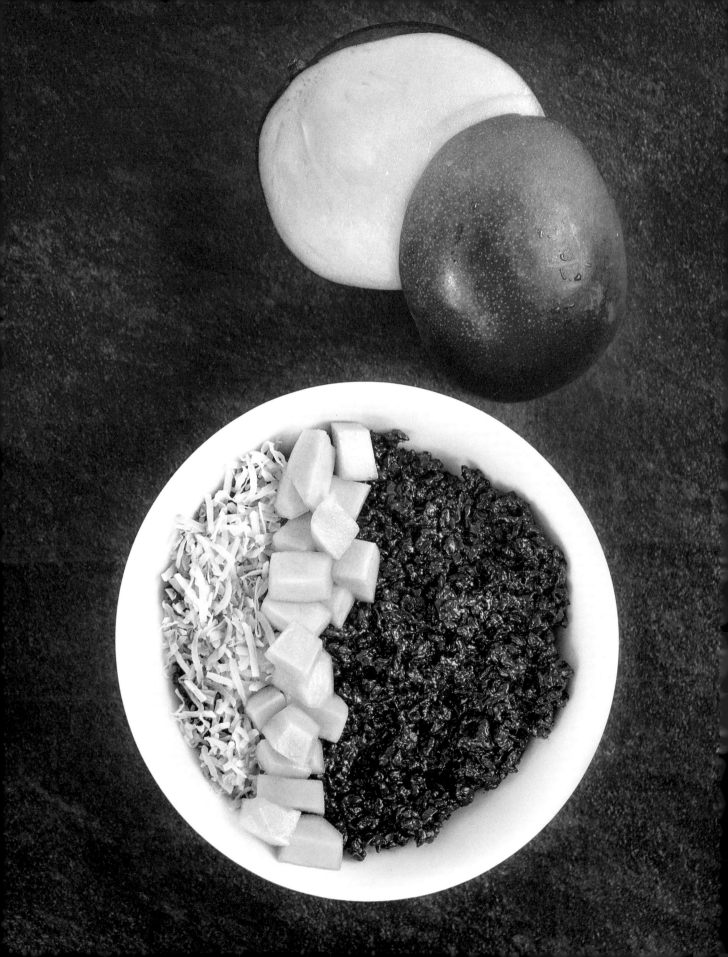

Coconut Forbidden Rice Pudding

The black rice in this breakfast pudding has loads of antioxidants and can help reduce histamine release and inflammation. The rice naturally contains anthocyanin, a flavonoid that provides the beautiful purple color.

····· SUPERFOOD · VEGAN ·····

PREP TIME: 5 minutes · COOK TIME: 45 minutes · TOTAL TIME: 50 minutes

1 cup black (forbidden) rice

2 (13½ ounce) cans coconut milk, divided

¼ cup coconut sugar

1 pinch salt

¼ cup shredded coconut (unsulfured, no preservatives, unsweetened)

1 mango, peeled, pitted, and sliced

1. In a medium saucepan, add the rice, 1½ cans (about 20 ounces) of coconut milk. Bring to a boil over medium-high heat. Reduce the heat to low and simmer, stirring occasionally, for 40 minutes or until the rice becomes tender.

2. Once the rice has cooked completely, add the remaining ½ can (about 6 ounces) of coconut milk, coconut sugar, and salt. Continue to cook, stirring until the mixture becomes thick and creamy.

3. In a skillet over medium heat, toast the coconut shreds—stirring constantly—for about 3 minutes or until they turn golden brown.

4. Serve the pudding warm, topped with the toasted coconut and fresh mango.

Tip

Make a big batch of this and freeze it in single-serving containers for 1–2 months. Thaw it for when you want a quick, healthy breakfast.

Variation

Top this delicious dish with other anti-inflammatory fruits, such as peaches or pears.

Crepes with Blueberries & Whipped Cream

Skinny pancakes, as they're known in my house, can work for pretty much any meal. You can use them as wraps for sandwiches because—don't forget!—you can fill them with savory foods, too, such as roasted butternut squash and onions topped with a drizzle of maple syrup. You can use the batter right away, but it thickens nicely while sitting in the fridge for two hours or overnight. Add a little more milk or water if the batter becomes too thick to make a skinny pancake.

····· CROWD PLEASER · LOW FODMAP · VEGETARIAN ·····

PREP TIME: 2 hours 30 minutes • COOK TIME: 10 minutes • TOTAL TIME: 2 hours 40 minutes

⅔ cups rolled oats

1 cup All-Purpose Flour Blend (page 28)

1 egg

1 cup milk of choice

½ cup water

3 tablespoons melted butter or extra-light virgin olive oil

1 pinch salt

1 pint fresh blueberries or other anti-inflammatory fruit

Whipped Cream or Whipped Coconut Cream (recipes follow)

Tip

Freeze the crepes in resealable freezer bags, separated by sheets of parchment paper, for up to 2 months.

1. In a food processor, pulse the rolled oats into ½ cup of oat flour.

2. In a medium mixing bowl, combine the oat flour, All-Purpose Flour Blend, egg, milk, water, melted butter, and salt. Whisk together until well incorporated and no lumps remain.

3. Chill in the refrigerator, covered, for 2 hours or overnight.

4. Preheat a small skillet over medium heat. When the skillet is hot, coat it with a little butter or oil, then add a ladleful of batter. Use the ladle to spread the batter around the skillet evenly. Cook for about 3 minutes, then carefully flip the crepe and continue cooking for 2–3 minutes on the remaining side.

5. Fold the crepe in quarters. Top with fresh fruit and Whipped Cream or Whipped Coconut Cream (recipes follow), roll them together, and top with more fruit and whipped cream.

WHIPPED CREAM

½ cup whipping cream
1 tablespoon maple syrup
½ teaspoon vanilla extract

1. In the bowl of a stand mixer, add the whipping cream. Using the whisk attachment, whip it on medium until the cream starts to stiffen.

2. Add the maple syrup and vanilla extract and continue whipping until stiff peaks form.

WHIPPED COCONUT CREAM

1 (13½ ounce) can coconut cream (refrigerated for 24 hours)
1 tablespoon maple syrup
½ teaspoon vanilla extract

In the bowl of a stand mixer, add the congealed coconut cream solids, maple syrup, and vanilla extract. Whip with the paddle attachment until they combine and become fluffy.

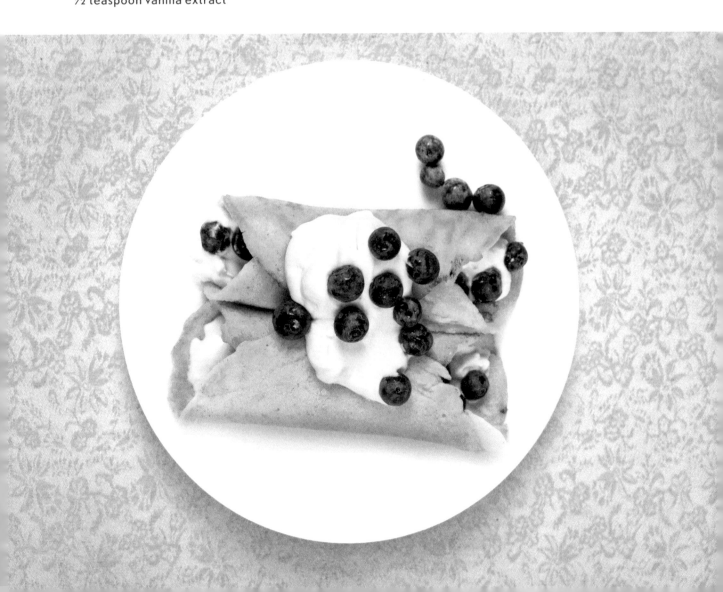

SNACKS

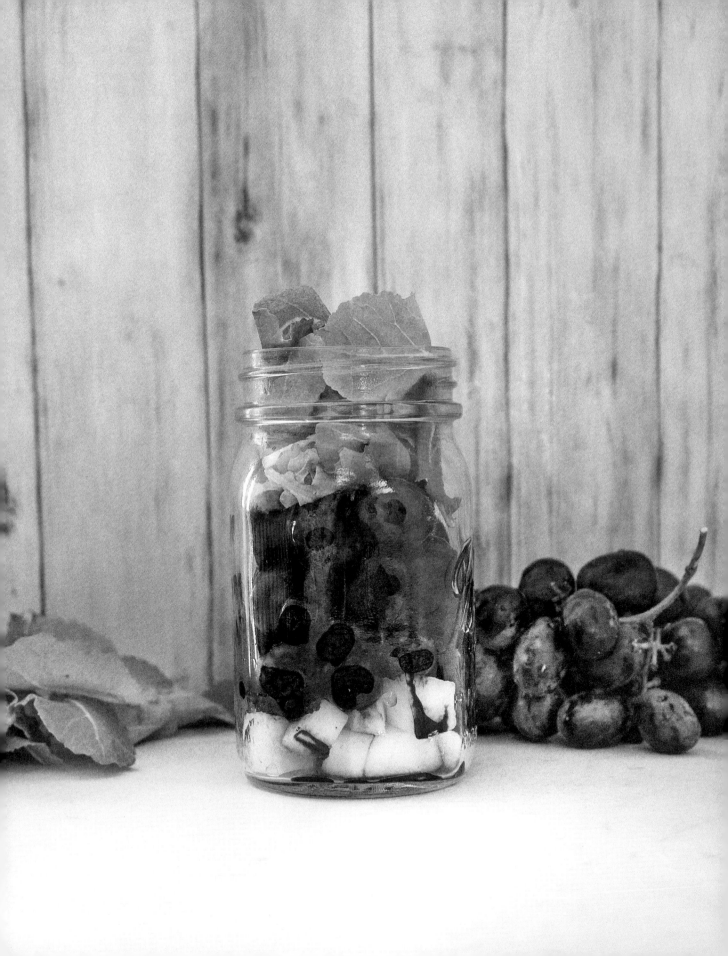

Deep Purple Smoothie

This smoothie contains tons of the dark flavonoids that act as powerful anti-inflammatory agents. It also provides lots of vitamin C and healthy fiber. Berry smoothies are a great way to sneak some green into your day, because the sweetness of the fruit easily masks the bitterness of the leafy greens.

····· FAST · GREAT SNACK · KID FRIENDLY · SUPERFOOD · VEGAN ·····

PREP TIME: 5 minutes • TOTAL TIME: 5 minutes

½ cup crushed ice

½ cup apple chunks

½ cup frozen blueberries

½ cup red or black grapes

¼ cup chopped fresh kale, stems removed

½ cup milk of choice

In a blender, add the ice, apples, blueberries, grapes, kale, and milk. Blend until smooth. Add more milk to taste if you want a thinner drink.

Tip

Smoothies can make great frozen treats for kids. Use a plastic mold or even just a small paper cup with a popsicle stick in the center of the smoothie mix and freeze. This is a great way to add natural, unsweetened fruit to your children's diet and hide some veggies in it—and they will think it's a treat!

Variation

For a lighter version of this recipe, substitute water for the milk.

Mango Coconut Smoothie

This smoothie is brimming with vitamins C and A. Ginger, an anti-inflammatory dynamo, gives it a spicy taste, but the creaminess of the coconut milk and the sweetness of the mango nicely mellow that. If you like spice, add more ginger to taste.

····· FAST · GREAT SNACK · SUPERFOOD · VEGAN ·····

PREP TIME: 5 minutes • TOTAL TIME: 5 minutes

1 cup frozen mango chunks
1 small carrot, diced
1 teaspoon grated ginger
⅓ cup coconut milk
¼ cup water

In a blender, add mango, carrot, ginger, coconut milk, and water. Blend until smooth.

Note

The coconut milk allows this recipe to freeze well. Pour into popsicle molds and freeze for a healthy treat.

Variation

Try substituting sweet potato for the carrot. It adds more creaminess to the smoothie but still provides a nice dose of vitamin A.

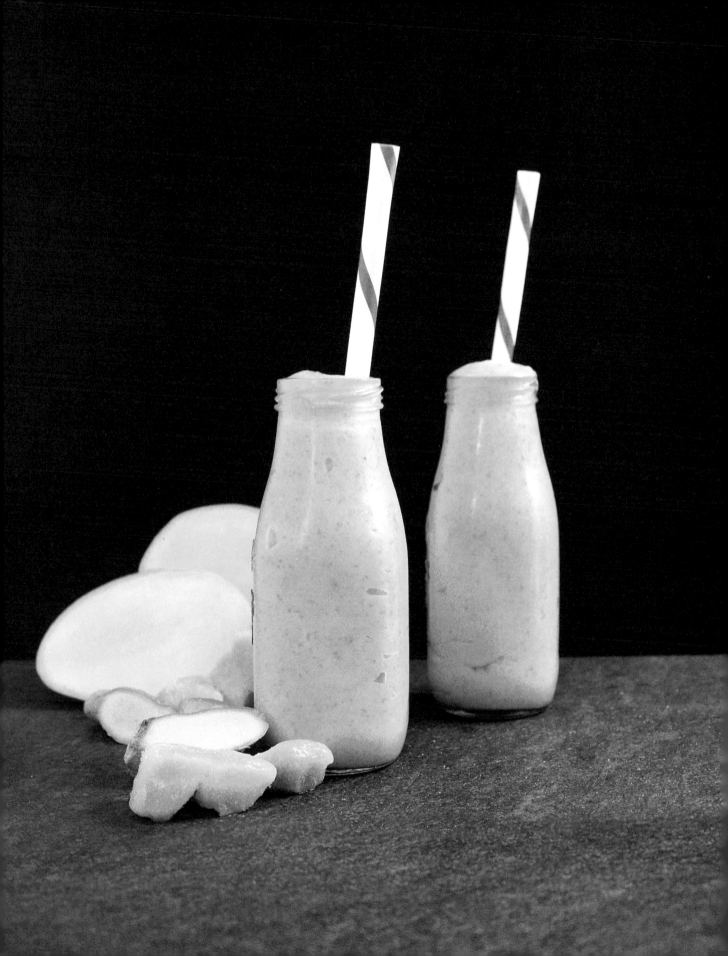

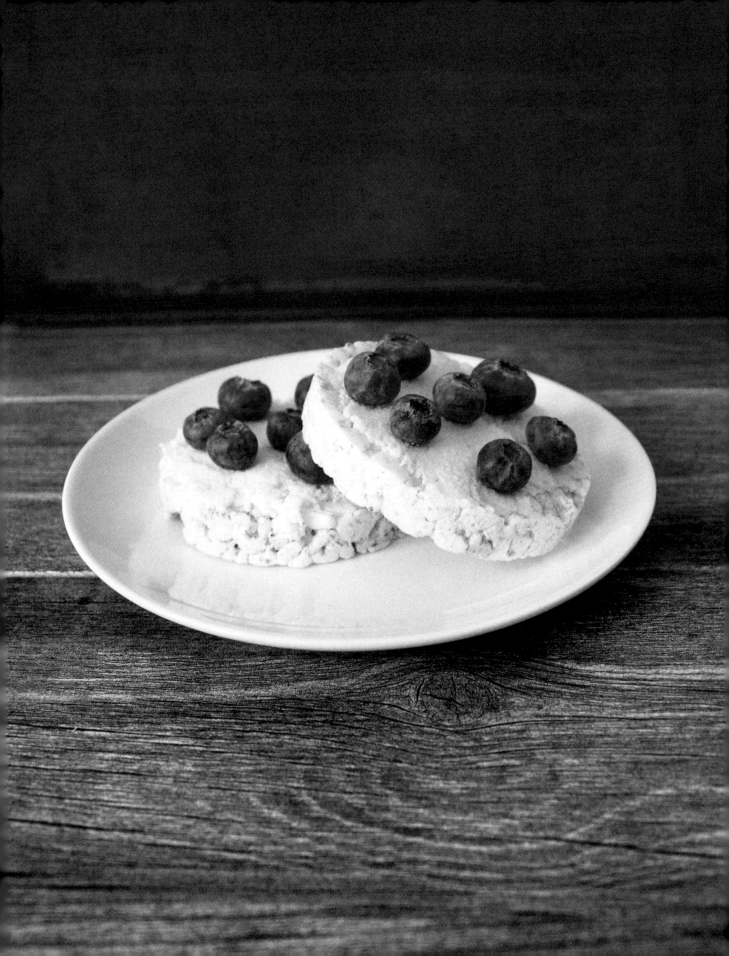

Rice Cakes with Coconut Butter & Fruit

Coconut butter makes a great substitute for nut or seed butters, so it's a great alternative for people with severe allergies. Many health food stores carry it, and you can spread it on bread or use it in the Crepes with Blueberries & Whipped Cream (page 62) instead of the whipped cream. With just a few pieces to assemble, this recipe is super quick, and the ingredients are basics that you always should have on hand. They also travel easily and don't require utensils or flatware to eat—just a knife to cut the fruit and then spread the butter. Consider this your go-to snack for your next picnic or road trip.

····· FAST · GREAT SNACK · LOW CAL · VEGAN ·····

PREP TIME: 5 minutes   •   TOTAL TIME: 5 minutes

2 brown rice cakes

2 tablespoons coconut butter (see below)

½ cup blueberries, mango chunks, or other fresh fruit

Top each rice cake with 1 tablespoon coconut butter and half of the fresh fruit.

Note

You can make your own coconut butter at home easily. In a food processor, add unsulfured, unsweetened coconut and pulse it until it becomes the consistency of butter. That's it! It will keep in the refrigerator for up to 1 week, or you can freeze it in ice cube trays and defrost it in the microwave before using. It will harden in the refrigerator so you will need to warm it up prior to spreading.

Variation

Take this recipe one step farther and transform it into a coconut butter and blueberry jam sandwich, like an anti-inflammatory PB&J.

Maple Sugar Popcorn

This variation is similar to kettle corn but with healthier coconut oil and maple sugar. It's also particularly good as a light offering for holiday parties at the end of the year.

····· FAST · GREAT SNACK · KID FRIENDLY · VEGAN ·····
PREP TIME: 5 minutes • COOK TIME: 5 minutes • TOTAL TIME: 10 minutes

¼ cup organic popping corn
    kernels
2 tablespoons coconut oil
1 tablespoon maple sugar
½ teaspoon salt

1. Using an air popper, make the popcorn according to the manufacturer's instructions.

2. In a microwave-safe bowl, melt the coconut oil by microwaving it on high for 30 seconds.

3. Add the maple sugar and salt to the oil and stir thoroughly.

4. Drizzle the oil mixture over the popcorn, mixing well to coat all of the pieces evenly, and serve immediately.

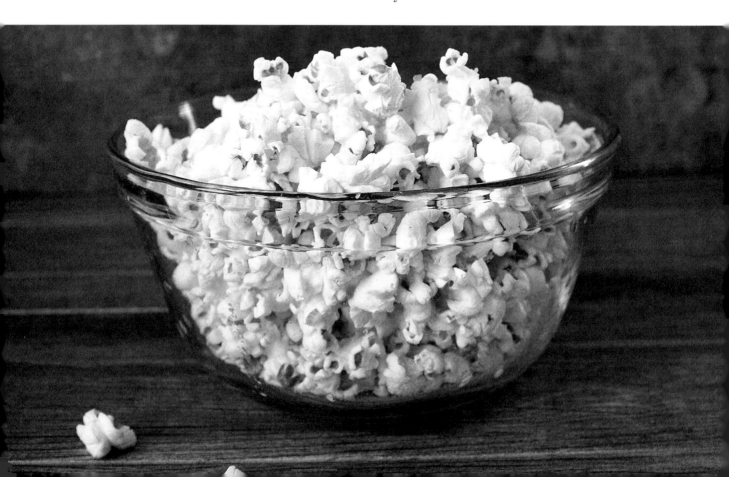

Herb Popcorn

Popcorn is a particularly healthy snack. It's a whole grain, and the herbs in this recipe add a big burst of taste as well as a nice boost of antioxidants. Make this handy snack for your next TV binge session or a party with friends.

····· CROWD PLEASER · FAST · GREAT SNACK · LOW CAL · VEGAN ·····

PREP TIME: 10 minutes • COOK TIME: 5 minutes • TOTAL TIME: 15 minutes

2 tablespoons extra-light olive oil

1 clove garlic

1 tablespoon minced rosemary

½ teaspoon sea salt

¼ cup organic popping corn kernels

1. In a small bowl, mix the olive oil, whole garlic clove, rosemary, and salt. Let it sit for 10 minutes so the flavors infuse into the oil.

2. Using an air popper, make the popcorn according to the manufacturer's instructions. Put in a large bowl.

3. Drizzle the oil and herb mixture over the popcorn, toss well to coat all of the pieces evenly, and serve immediately.

Note

Infusing the olive oil with the fresh herbs distributes the flavor better, so let those and the garlic steep for at least 10 minutes before spreading over the popcorn.

Variation

Use your herbs of choice. Pick any fresh herbs from your garden or window box—basil, chives, dill, parsley—or use dried. Use 1 tablespoon for fresh and 1 teaspoon for dried. If using fresh, mince the leaves very small so the flavor distributes evenly.

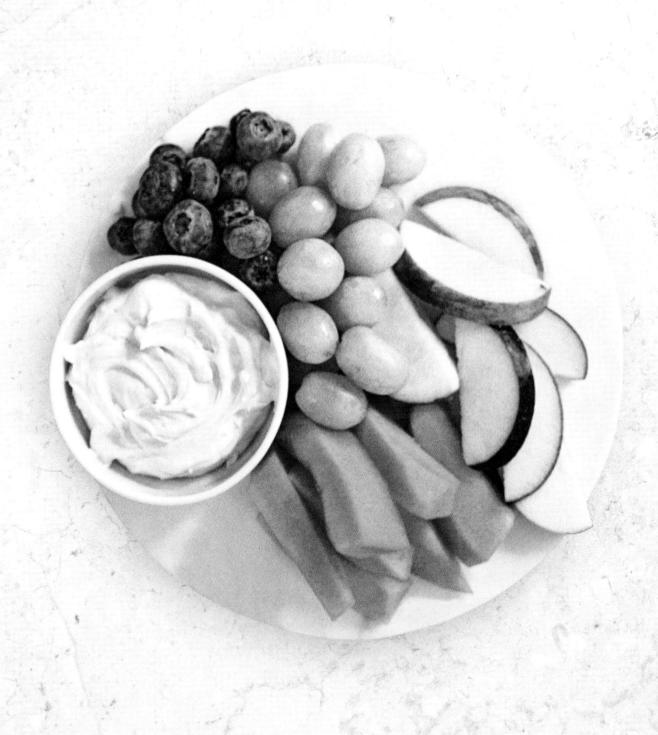

Fruit Plate with Whipped Coconut Cream

This recipe gives you a quick and easy way to make fruit a little more exciting. The whipped cream tastes decadent, but it's really a healthy, sweet treat. It also makes a good summer spread for picnics or parties.

····· CROWD PLEASER · FAST · GREAT SNACK · VEGAN ·····

PREP TIME: 15 minutes • TOTAL TIME: 15 minutes

1 (13½) ounce can coconut cream (refrigerated for 24 hours)
½ teaspoon vanilla extract
1 tablespoon maple syrup
1 cup blueberries
1 cup grapes
1 cup sliced apples
1 cup cantaloupe chunks

1. Open the can of coconut cream and carefully scoop the cream solids into the bowl of a stand mixer.

2. Using the paddle attachment, start whipping the coconut cream.

3. Add the vanilla extract and maple syrup. Whip for about 2 minutes until the cream becomes fluffy.

3. Serve the cream with fruit.

> ### Note
>
> *Eat more grapes! Studies have shown that grapes can reduce the risk of developing cancer and heart disease, and they decrease inflammation. All grapes have protective phytonutrients, so enjoy the green, red, or black varieties—whichever you prefer.*
>
> ### Tip
>
> *If the fruit plate is going to sit out for a little bit, brush a few drops of lemon juice onto the apples to prevent them from turning brown.*
>
> ### Variation
>
> *If you can't find coconut cream, refrigerate a can of coconut milk overnight or, better yet, for 24 hours. When you open it, the cream will have hardened at the top. You may need to use several cans of coconut milk to attain the same amount of solids as you get from a can of coconut cream.*

Melon Cooler

On a hot summer day, nothing tastes better than some cool, refreshing melon. This recipe blends three different melons with crushed ice for a cooling and hydrating treat packed with loads of vitamin C.

····· FAST · GREAT SNACK · KID FRIENDLY · LOW CAL · SUPERFOOD · VEGAN ·····

PREP TIME: **15 minutes** • TOTAL TIME: **15 minutes**

1½ cups crushed ice, divided
1 cup honeydew chunks
1 cup watermelon chunks
1 cup cantaloupe chunks

1. In a blender, add ½ cup crushed ice and the honeydew chunks and blend until frothy. Divide evenly into 2 glasses.

2. Repeat step 1 with the watermelon chunks. Divide evenly on top of the honeydew, pouring the mixture over a spoon to help the layer spread evenly.

3. Repeat step 1 with the cantaloupe chunks. Divide evenly on top of the watermelon.

4. Garnish with melon chunks of choice, and serve with a straw to enjoy one layer at a time.

Variation

This recipe works well with other fruits if you remove the skins. Try using mangos and peaches as well. These fruits contain less water than melons, so add extra water when blending to make sure they come out perfectly smooth.

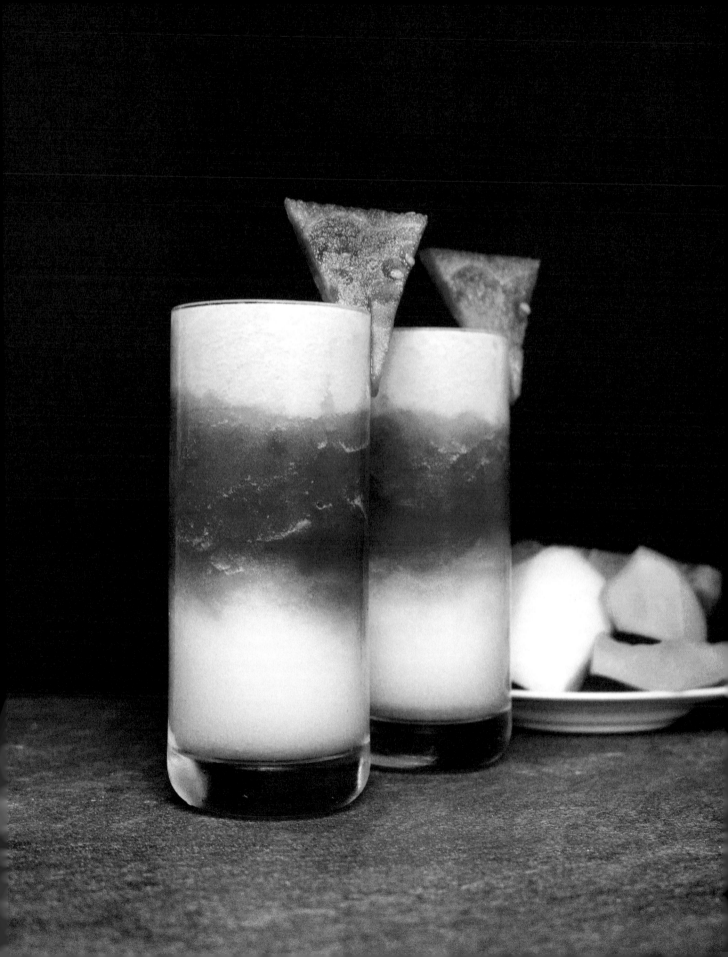

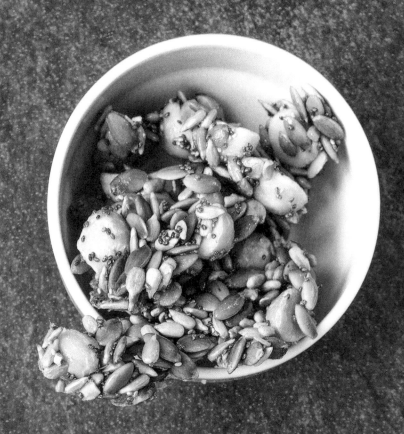

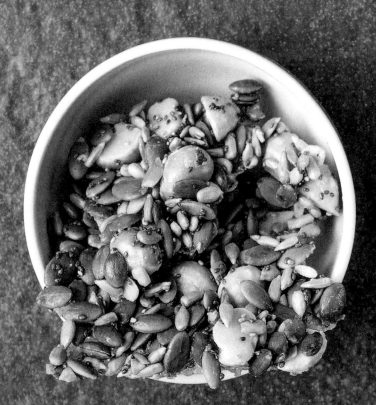

Macadamia Nut Crunch

Seeds and nuts form a key component of a well-balanced diet in general and the anti-inflammatory diet in particular. Some nuts—such as almonds, cashews, pecans, and walnuts—have high levels of histamine, so we're avoiding those in favor of macadamia nuts, which have lower levels. This yummy nut crunch has a touch of sweetness from the maple syrup and boasts large amounts of vitamin E, good fats, minerals, omega-3s, and protein. Pack some for your next walk or hike.

····· GREAT SNACK · HIGH PROTEIN · KID FRIENDLY · SUPERFOOD · VEGAN ·····
PREP TIME: 5 minutes • COOK TIME: 20 minutes • TOTAL TIME: 25 minutes

1 cup raw macadamia nuts

1 cup raw pumpkin seeds

1 cup raw sunflower seeds

2 tablespoons chia seeds

2 tablespoons maple syrup

½ teaspoon salt

1. Preheat the oven to 350°F.

2. Line a baking sheet with parchment paper.

3. In a mixing bowl, combine the nuts, seeds, maple syrup, and salt. Stir to combine thoroughly.

4. Spread the nut mixture evenly onto the paper-lined sheet.

5. Bake for 15–20 minutes or until golden. Let cool and break into pieces for a healthy snack.

Tip
Freeze in airtight single-serving containers or resealable freezer bags for up to 3 months.

Variation
Crumble this crunch into a granola and have it with milk as a breakfast cereal or mix it with coconut cream for a low-histamine version of yogurt and granola. You can also use it as a salad topper instead of croutons.

Oat Crackers

These amazing crackers taste better than the gluten-free crackers that you can buy in most grocery stores. The herbs give them lots of rosmarinic acid, which stabilizes mast cells, and the oats provide fiber and protein.

····· GREAT SNACK · VEGAN ·····

PREP TIME: 10 minutes • COOK TIME: 35 minutes • TOTAL TIME: 45 minutes

2 cups rolled oats

1/3 cup All-Purpose Flour Blend (page 28)

½ teaspoon salt, divided

½ teaspoon baking powder

1 tablespoon chopped herbs or spices of choice (chives, parsley, rosemary, thyme, etc.)

3 tablespoons olive oil, divided

1. Preheat the oven to 350°F.

2. Line a baking sheet with parchment paper.

3. In a food processor, pulse the rolled oats into 1½ cups oat flour.

4. In a mixing bowl, combine the oat flour, All-Purpose Flour Blend, ¼ teaspoon salt, baking powder, herbs, 2 tablespoons of the olive oil, and ¼ cup water into a dough.

5. Knead the dough together lightly for 1–2 minutes. Add a little extra water if it feels too dry.

6. Drizzle 1 tablespoon of olive oil on the parchment paper to cover the surface where you will roll out the dough.

7. Place the dough on parchment paper and roll it out to ¼-inch thickness.

8. Using a pizza cutter, slice the dough into 1½-inch squares and cut off the rough edges. Make fork holes in the crackers if desired and sprinkle with the remaining salt.

9. Bake for 35 minutes or until crispy.

Variation

Try basil, black cumin, cardamom, cumin, dill, garlic, oregano, or sage solo or mix and match your favorites. For plain crackers, simply omit the herbs or spices.

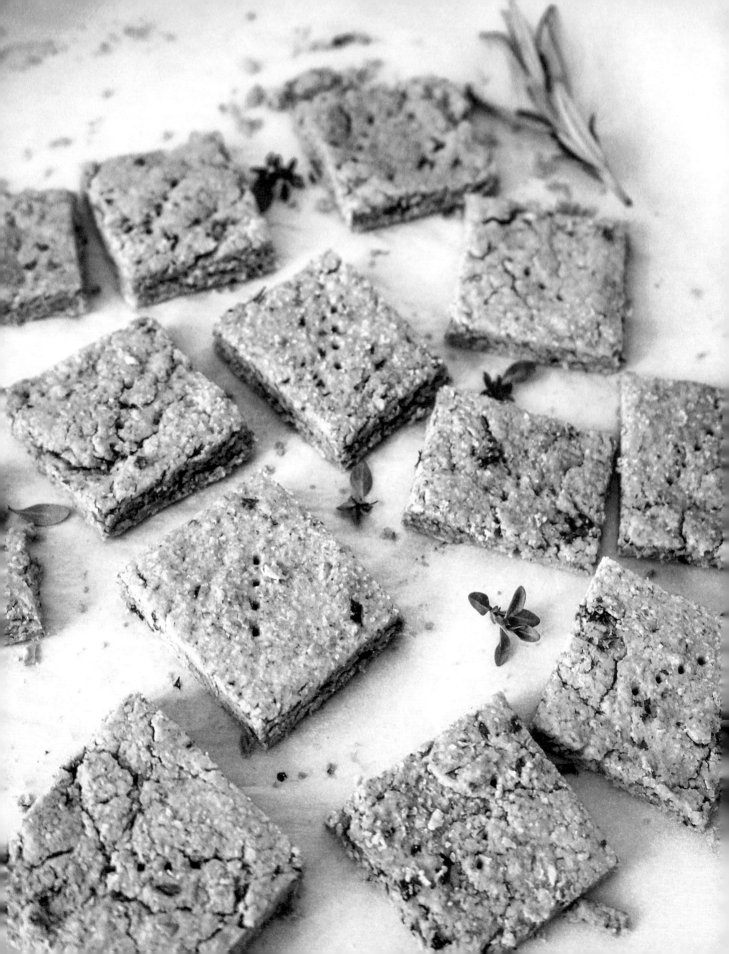

LUNCH

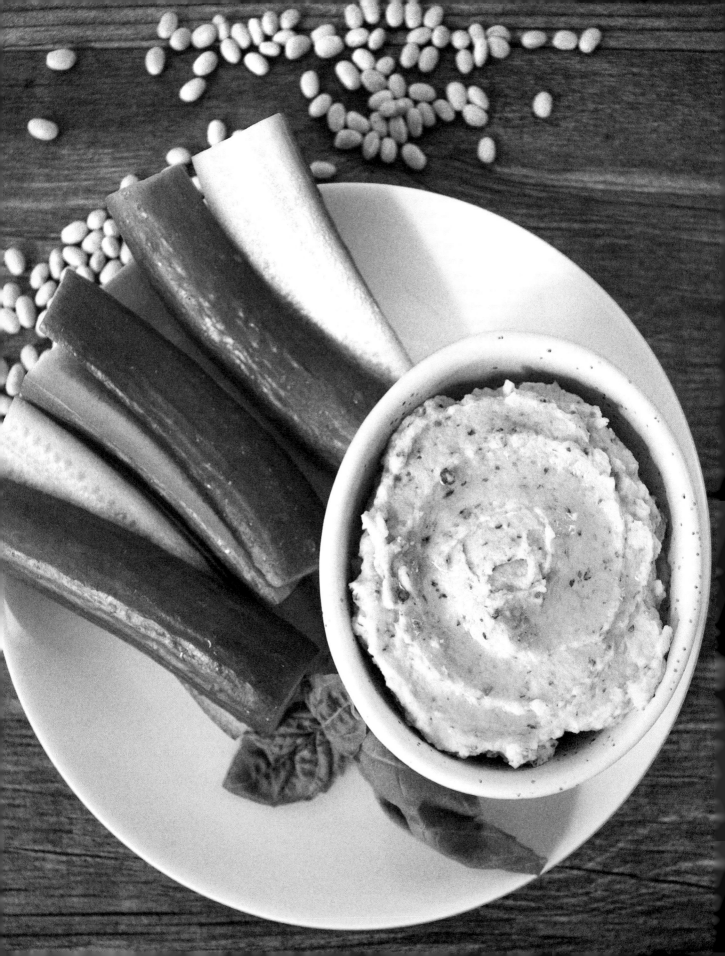

White Bean & Basil Dip

This is a delicious, summery way to enjoy a hummus-like dip. The white beans offer a great source of plant-based protein, and they blend into a creamy puree. The basil and garlic provide antioxidants to reduce inflammation. Make a batch or two, freeze in an ice cube tray, then thaw as needed for a quick snack or a sandwich or wrap spread.

····· CROWD PLEASER · FAST · GREAT SNACK · HIGH PROTEIN · VEGAN ·····

PREP TIME: 10 minutes • TOTAL TIME: 10 minutes

2 cups white beans, cooked from dry or thawed
2 cloves garlic
2 cups fresh basil leaves
¼ cup extra-virgin olive oil
juice of ½ lemon
1 pinch salt

Into the bowl of a food processor, add all ingredients and puree until smooth.

Note

You can use navy, cannellini, or great northern beans for this recipe. Try making batches of each to see which you like best.

To cook the beans from dry, add the dry beans to a bowl, cover with water, and soak for 8 hours. Drain and rinse the beans and cover with water in a pan. Over medium heat, boil them for about 30 minutes. Test to make sure they're tender, then drain, rinse, and freeze the beans in freezer bags.

Tip

This dip makes a great snack when paired with rice crackers or raw veggies. For a super-quick and easy lunch, add a serving to an Oat-Flour Wrap with the veggies of your choice.

Super Salad with Sesame Garlic Dressing

This powerhouse salad will give your body great big doses of vitamin C, magnesium, vitamin A, and anti-inflammatory phytonutrients along with an immune-system boost. The sesame seeds in the dressing add a creamy and nutty taste to the dish.

····· FAST · LOW CAL · SUPERFOOD · VEGAN ·····

PREP TIME: 15 minutes • TOTAL TIME: 15 minutes

1 large head lettuce

2 carrots

1 red bell pepper

1 cup sliced purple cabbage

¼ cup raw pumpkin seeds

sesame seeds for garnish

Sesame Garlic Dressing
    (page 235)

1. Chop the lettuce, shred the carrots, and slice the bell pepper.

2. In a large bowl, combine lettuce, carrots, pepper, cabbage, and pumpkin seeds.

3. Toss dressing with salad and garnish with sesame seeds.

> **Note**
>
> *Use your lettuce of choice. I recommend romaine, red leaf, or endive for this recipe.*

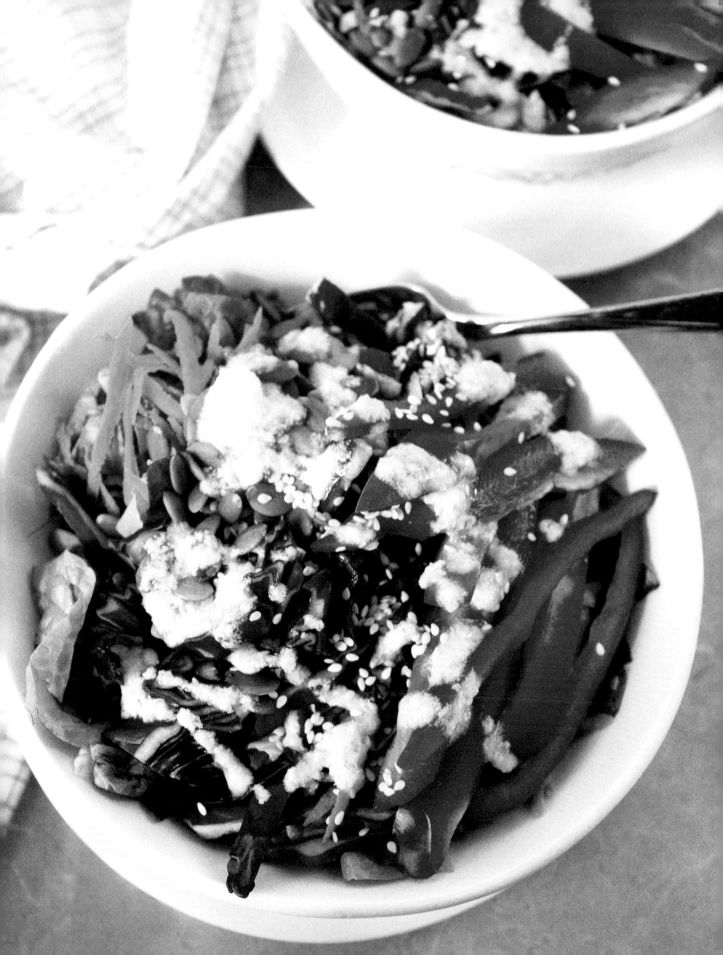

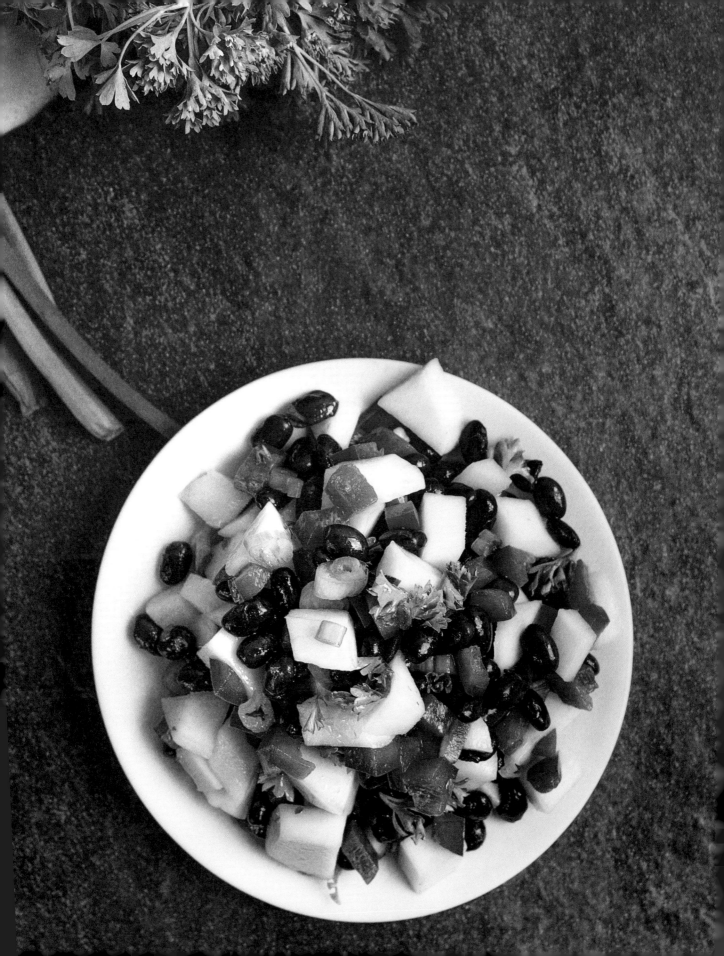

Mango Bean Salad

The black beans in this salad provide anthocyanin, an antioxidant and the same flavonoid in black rice and blueberries. It also boasts a bunch of vitamin C from the mango and red bell pepper, both of which liven up the earthiness of the beans. It tastes great on its own, particularly as a vivid healthy option for a summer picnic, but also try it as salsa for corn chips or with grilled chicken or salmon.

CROWD PLEASER · FAST · HIGH PROTEIN · SUPERFOOD · VEGAN

PREP TIME: 15 minutes　•　TOTAL TIME: 15 minutes

1 mango
1 cup black beans (cooked from dry or thawed)
½ red bell pepper, chopped
2 scallions, chopped
juice of ½ lemon or lime
salt and pepper

1. Peel, pit, and dice the mango.

2. In a medium bowl, add all the ingredients and stir to combine thoroughly.

3. Divide into individual servings and enjoy.

> **Note**
>
> *If you eat this dish with corn chips, choose organic to reduce your intake of pesticides and GMOs—or make your own corn chips at home from the Corn Tortillas (page 101).*

Loaded Greek Salad

This salad is brimming with oregano and onion, both potent anti-inflammatory agents that reduce histamine release. Having a salad a day is a great way to stick to an anti-inflammatory eating habit. A serving of this salad provides three servings of veggies, a third of your daily recommended intake, so chomp on this one often.

····· FAST · LOW CAL · SUPERFOOD · VEGAN ·····

PREP TIME: 15 minutes • TOTAL TIME: 15 minutes

2 carrots

1 cucumber

½ red onion

1 red pepper sliced in
⅓-inch strips

1 cup chickpeas (cooked
from dry or thawed)

8 cups mesclun greens

DRESSING

1 tablespoon minced red
onion

4 tablespoons extra-virgin
olive oil

juice of 1 lemon

1 tablespoon dried oregano

½ teaspoon salt

1. Shred the carrots, slice the cucumber, and peel and slice the onion.

2. Add them and the sliced pepper to a large bowl with the beans and greens.

3. To make the dressing, in a small bowl, combine the minced onion, olive oil, lemon juice, oregano, and salt and whisk together.

4. Toss the salad with the dressing if eating it right away.

> **Note**
>
> *Keeping the beans frozen until you're ready to eat them reduces spoilage, so consider prepping the vegetables for 2–3 salads and defrosting the chickpeas right before mixing the salad with the dressing.*
>
> **Tip**
>
> *If you're taking this salad with you to work or on a trip, pack the veggies in a large container and the dressing in a separate container. Dress the salad just before mealtime.*

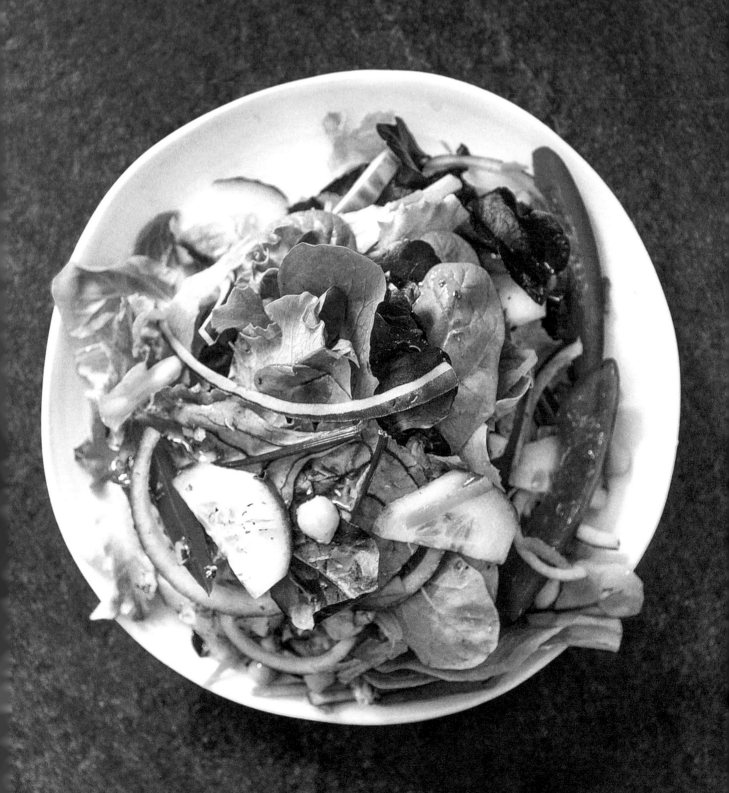

Roasted Asparagus with Fried Eggs & Pea Shoots

Eggs are great for breakfast, but they're a great source of protein and omega-3s, so why stop there? Have some for lunch! Pea shoots are one of the few sources of natural DAO, the enzyme that breaks down histamine, and asparagus provides an amazing source of antioxidants and quercetin, containing nearly as much as onions. Asparagus also contains lots of vitamin K and folate. This nutrient-dense meal works well any time of the day. It looks elegant but couldn't be simpler.

····· DAIRY FREE · LOW CAL · SUPERFOOD · VEGETARIAN ·····

PREP TIME: **5** minutes • COOK TIME: **15** minutes • TOTAL TIME: **20** minutes

1 bunch asparagus, woody
    stems removed
1 teaspoon extra-light olive
    oil, plus 1 tablespoon for
    frying
½ teaspoon salt, divided
4 eggs
1 cup pea shoots
    (see below)

1. Preheat oven to 375°F.

2. Toss asparagus in 1 teaspoon olive oil and a pinch of salt, coating evenly.

3. Place on a baking sheet and roast for about 10 minutes or until browned.

4. In a skillet over medium heat, add 1 tablespoon of olive oil and then the eggs. Cook until the whites set, about 2 minutes.

5. Flip the eggs and cook for 1–2 more minutes depending on whether you like a runnier or firmer yolk.

6. Layer the eggs over the roasted asparagus and top with fresh pea shoots, a drizzle of olive oil, and salt to taste.

> **Note**
>
> *You can buy pea shoots at most grocery stores, or you can grow them, indoors or outside, from pea seeds.*

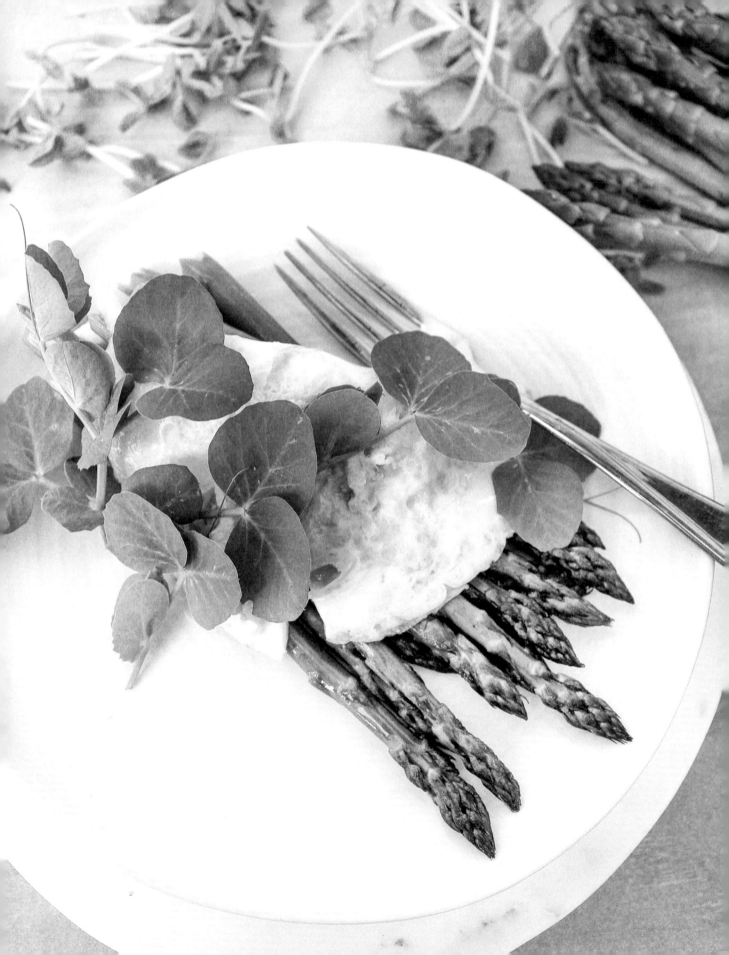

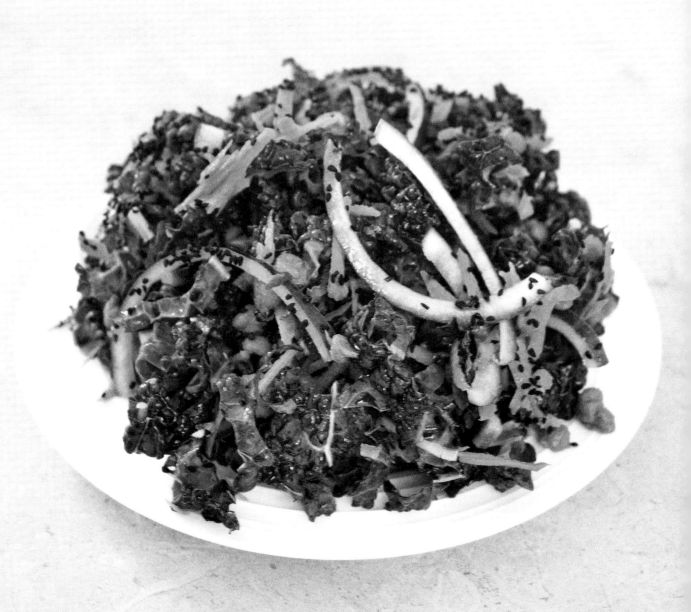

Carrot, Lentil & Kale Salad

Indian cooking often uses black cumin, also known as black seed or *Nigella sativa*, which has some of the most powerful anti-inflammatory and antihistamine properties of any spice. The lentils give this super-healthy salad some added protein power, and the kale helps with detoxification and provides lots of vitamins A and C. Lacinato kale—the flat one also known as Tuscan kale or dinosaur kale—is a little sweeter than its curly cousin, so you may prefer it to more bitter kinds of kale that you've tried before. Make sure to remove the stem and central vein before chopping the kale.

····· SUPERFOOD · VEGAN ·····

PREP TIME: 20 minutes • TOTAL TIME: 20 minutes

4 cups lacinato kale, cleaned and stems removed

2 carrots

2 cups cooked lentils

½ red onion

1 teaspoon black cumin *(Nigella sativa)* for garnish

DRESSING

1 tablespoon minced red onion

4 tablespoons extra-virgin olive oil

½ teaspoon salt

juice of ½ lemon

½ teaspoon cumin

1. Finely chop the kale and place in a large bowl.

2. Shred the carrots and add them to the bowl along with the lentils.

3. Cut the onion into ¼-inch thick slices and add to the bowl as well.

4. To make the dressing, in a small bowl, combine the minced red onion, olive oil, salt, lemon juice, and cumin. Stir thoroughly to combine.

5. Toss the salad with the dressing gently to avoid breaking the lentils.

6. Garnish with black cumin.

> **Tip**
>
> *This salad makes a great filling for an oat wrap for a quick vegan snack or lunch.*

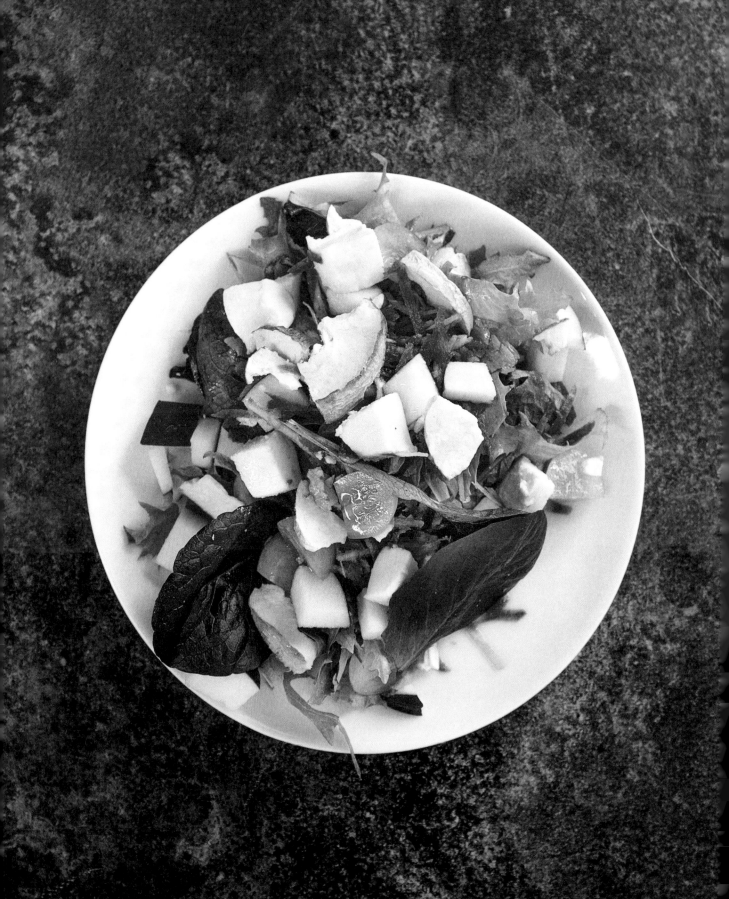

Sweet & Savory Salad

The heaps of antioxidants in this salad come from its purple carrots, grapes, and apples. Resveratrol from grapes and quercetin from apples help reduce histamine release and lower inflammation. You can omit the mozzarella cheese if you need or want to, but it's one of the few cheeses allowed on the anti-inflammatory, low-histamine diet, and it nicely balances the sweetness of the fruit, so enjoy it in moderation.

····· LOW CAL · SUPERFOOD · VEGETARIAN ·····

PREP TIME: 20 minutes • TOTAL TIME: 20 minutes

1 red apple

juice of 1 lemon

8 cups chopped romaine lettuce or mixed greens

1 cup red or green grapes, halved

2 purple carrots, shredded

1 (4-ounce) ball fresh mozzarella cheese

1 cup freeze-dried apple chips for garnish

DRESSING

juice of 1 lemon

2 tablespoons apple juice

¼ cup extra-virgin olive oil

1 tablespoon maple syrup

½ teaspoon salt

1. Core the apple and cut it into ¼-inch slices.

2. Brush the slices in lemon juice to prevent browning.

3. In a large bowl, combine the lettuce, grapes, apples, carrots, and cheese.

4. To make the dressing, in a small bowl, whisk the lemon juice, apple juice, olive oil, and maple syrup together.

5. Add the salt to the dressing and stir to dissolve.

6. Toss the dressing with the salad and garnish with freeze-dried apples.

Beet & Sweet Potato Rösti

A rösti is a potato fritter often eaten for breakfast in Switzerland, but this version—really a more nutrient-packed latke sans potato—eats more like lunch. The sweet potato and beets provide ample phytonutrients, vitamins A and C, and lots of fiber. They also have lower levels of carbohydrates than potato pancakes. Think of this dish as your new elevated hash browns.

····· CROWD PLEASER · DAIRY FREE · GREAT SNACK · SUPERFOOD · VEGETARIAN ·····

PREP TIME: 5 minutes · COOK TIME: 20 minutes · TOTAL TIME: 25 minutes

1 large beet

1 sweet potato

1 onion

1 egg

2 tablespoons tapioca starch

½ teaspoon salt

4 tablespoons extra-light olive oil, divided

Tip

Make a couple of batches of these and freeze them in resealable freezer bags for up to 3 months. Then, for a quick lunch or breakfast, simply reheat one in a toaster oven at 375°F for about 10 minutes.

1. Preheat oven to 400°F.

2. Drizzle 1 tablespoon olive oil onto a baking sheet and set aside.

3. Peel and shred the beet, sweet potato, and onion. A food processor will do the job quickly.

4. In a large bowl, combine the shredded beet, sweet potato, and onion and add the egg, tapioca starch, and salt.

5. In a large pan, over medium heat, add 2 tablespoons of olive oil.

6. Drop the rösti batter, ¼ cup at a time, into the pan. Let cook for about 5–6 minutes, until golden on the bottom.

7. Drizzle the tops of the röstis with 1 tablespoon olive oil to prevent sticking when flipping. Flip the röstis and cook on the other side for 5 more minutes.

8. Transfer the röstis to the prepared baking sheet and bake for 5–10 minutes, until extra crispy.

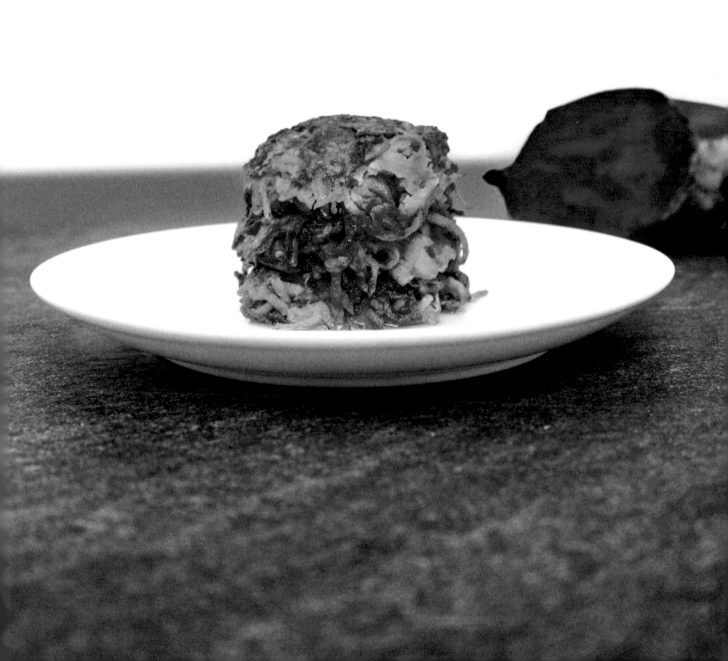

Oat-Flour Wraps

This oat wrap gives you a nice option for holding hummus and veggies or as a base for flatbread pizza. The oats provide protein and fiber, and the tapioca starch helps it all stick together yet remain flexible.

····· GREAT SNACK · VEGAN ·····

PREP TIME: 10 minutes • COOK TIME: 15 minutes • TOTAL TIME: 25 minutes

2 cups rolled oats

2 tablespoons ground chia seeds

$\frac{2}{3}$ cup tapioca starch

$\frac{1}{2}$ cup hot water

$\frac{1}{4}$ cup extra-light olive oil, plus more for cooking

$\frac{1}{2}$ teaspoon salt

1. In a food processor, pulse the oats into 1½ cups of oat flour.

2. Combine all of the ingredients and mix together until a dough forms. Add a little more water if necessary for the dough to stick together properly.

3. Divide the dough into 4 balls.

4. Using a tortilla press or rolling pin, dust the surface with tapioca starch and press out each dough ball to an ⅛-inch thickness. Or put the dough ball between two pieces of parchment paper and roll out to a thin circle.

5. In a skillet over medium heat, drizzle a little olive oil and place the wrap in the pan. Cook for 1–2 minutes or until golden. Flip and cook on the other side for another 1–2 minutes.

6. Repeat with remaining wraps.

> **Tip**
>
> *Freeze the wraps between parchment paper in a resealable freezer bag for up to 3 months, then reheat them for quick meals.*
>
> **Variation**
>
> *Add garlic or herbs to the dough when mixing to make wraps with some extra zing. It will give your veggie wraps a tasty boost of flavor.*

Corn Tortillas

Confession: I'm not a great tortilla maker. My corn tortillas struggled to stay together until experimentation prompted me to add some tapioca starch to the mix, which helped a lot. That secret ingredient allows the tortilla to flex more and be more forgiving to us novice tortilla-making cooks.

····· GREAT SNACK · VEGAN ·····

PREP TIME: 10 minutes • COOK TIME: 25 minutes • TOTAL TIME: 35 minutes

2 cups masa harina
  (corn flour)
⅔ cup tapioca starch
2 tablespoons extra-light
  olive oil
1 cup hot water
1 pinch salt

Tip

Freeze the tortillas, with parchment paper between them, in a resealable freezer bag, for up to 3 months. Then reheat one or more for a quick wrap for hummus and veggies or fajitas.

Variation

Use this recipe to make corn chips, too! In a small pan over medium heat, add 2 tablespoons extra-light olive oil. Add the tortilla and cook for about 2–3 minutes per side, until crispy. Use a pizza cutter to slice it into strips or chips.

1. In a medium bowl, combine all the ingredients until a dough forms. Add a little more water if needed.

2. Divide the dough into 8 balls.

3. Let the dough rest, covered with a towel, for 10 minutes.

4. Using a tortilla press or parchment paper, press or roll each ball to an ⅛-inch thickness. If using a tortilla press, sprinkle each side of the press with some masa harina so the dough won't stick.

5. In a medium skillet over medium heat, dry-cook 1 tortilla at a time for about 90 seconds or until golden on the bottom.

6. Flip and cook on the other side for about 90 seconds. Cool before handling.

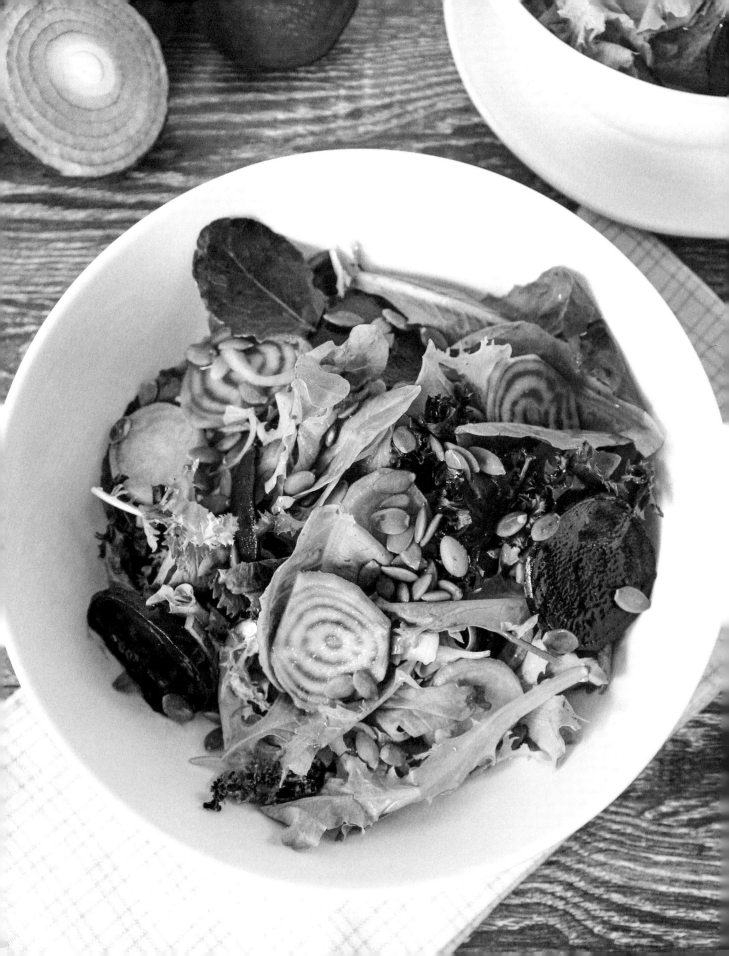

Beets & Greens Salad

Beets are one of nature's most amazing anti-inflammatory superfoods. They contain loads of antioxidants, they can help lower your blood pressure, and they have lots of fiber. Using different colors of beets creates a feast for the eyes. Different beets also have slight variations in taste. Chioggia beets, which are pink striped, and golden beets work particularly well.

····· LOW CAL · SUPERFOOD · VEGAN ·····

PREP TIME: 10 minutes • COOK TIME: 20 minutes • TOTAL TIME: 30 minutes

8 cups mixed greens

1 red beet

1 chioggia or candy-striped beet

1 golden beet

3 tablespoons olive oil, divided

2 tablespoons maple syrup

juice of ½ lemon

1 pinch salt

½ cup raw pumpkin seeds

1. Preheat the oven to 350°F.

2. Peel the beets and slice into them into ¼-inch rounds.

3. Toss the beets with 1 tablespoon of olive oil and place them on a baking sheet.

4. Bake for 15–20 minutes, until fork tender.

5. Prepare dressing by combining 2 tablespoons olive oil, maple syrup, lemon juice, and salt in a small dish.

6. Add the greens to a large bowl, followed by the beets and pumpkin seeds.

7. Toss with the dressing.

Garlic Flatbread

This flatbread is crispier and has more of a rise than the Corn Tortillas (page 101). It also makes a nice base for pizza or a more hearty option for dipping in hummus or soups. The garlic adds lots of antioxidants and anti-inflammatory power.

····· GREAT SNACK · VEGAN ·····

PREP TIME: **10** minutes • COOK TIME: **20** minutes • TOTAL TIME: **30** minutes

1 ¼ cup All-Purpose Flour Blend (page 28)

1 cup rolled oats

2 tablespoons garlic oil (see below)

¾ cup milk of choice

1 teaspoon baking powder

¼ teaspoon salt

1 tablespoon olive oil for cooking

fresh herbs of choice: basil, chives, parsley, rosemary, thyme, etc.

3 tablespoons extra-light olive oil, divided, for frying

1. In a food processor, pulse the rolled oats into ¾ cup of oat flour.

2. In a bowl, combine the All-Purpose Flour Blend, oat flour, garlic oil, milk, baking powder, salt, and fresh herbs until they form a dough.

3. Divide the dough into 3 pieces and flatten each piece by hand to about ⅓-inch thickness.

4. In a medium skillet over medium heat, add 1 tablespoon olive oil and then 1 flatbread at a time. Cover the skillet with a lid for 2–3 minutes or until the dough turns golden.

5. Flip the flatbread, cover again, and cook for 2–3 more minutes. 2 the flatbread helps it to rise.

6. Repeat for the remaining flatbreads.

Note

For the garlic oil, steep crushed garlic in oil for 5 minutes before adding it to mix. Use both the crushed garlic and oil in the recipe. If you have IBS or IBD, let the whole clove steep in the oil and remove it just before mixing in the oil.

Tip

For a more filling meal, serve a flatbread alongside the Acorn Squash Soup (page 111), Kale & White Bean Soup (page 115), Roasted Carrot & Garlic Hummus (page 116), Superfood Stew (page 119), or White Bean & Basil Dip (page 85).

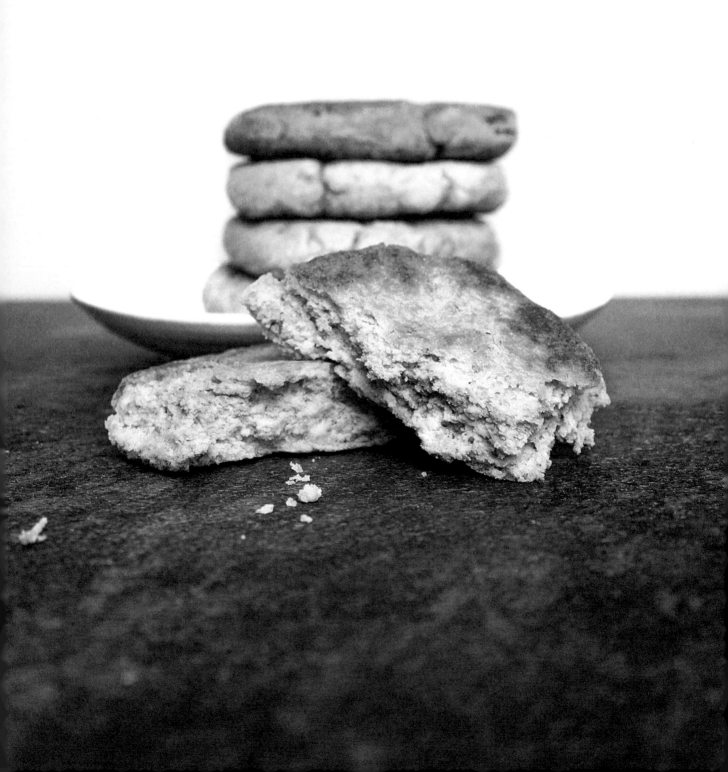

Quinoa, Beet & Corn Salad

As the beets color the quinoa, this salad takes on a beautiful pink hue (a useful point if you have a little one who likes unicorns). Quinoa is a naturally complete protein, so this meatless meal has great filling power because of its fiber and plant-protein content. Beets are a great anti-inflammatory food, and using tricolor quinoa will give you even more antioxidants.

····· HIGH PROTEIN · KID FRIENDLY · SUPERFOOD · VEGAN ·····

PREP TIME: **10** minutes • COOK TIME: **20** minutes • TOTAL TIME: **30** minutes

2 cups dry quinoa

4 cups water

3 beets

2 tablespoons olive oil, divided

1 cup organic corn (frozen or fresh off the cob)

2 tablespoons chopped chives

juice of 1 lemon

salt

1. In a pot over high heat, cook the quinoa in the water. When the water boils, reduce the heat to low and simmer for about 20 minutes or until all the liquid absorbs. Fluff with a fork and set aside.

2. Meanwhile, add the beets to a small pot and cover with water. Boil for about 10–15 minutes, until the beets are fork tender.

3. Rinse the beets with cold water and remove the skins, which should slide right off.

4. Chop the beets into ½-inch pieces.

5. In a skillet over medium heat, add 1 tablespoon olive oil and the corn. Sauté until the corn turns golden, about 3–4 minutes, which will bring out more of its flavor.

6. In a large bowl, combine the quinoa, beets, corn, and chives. Add olive oil, lemon juice to taste, and salt to taste. Stir to combine thoroughly.

Variation

You can enjoy this dish warm or cold, depending on the season and your preference. If it's in season, use fresh, organic sweet corn.

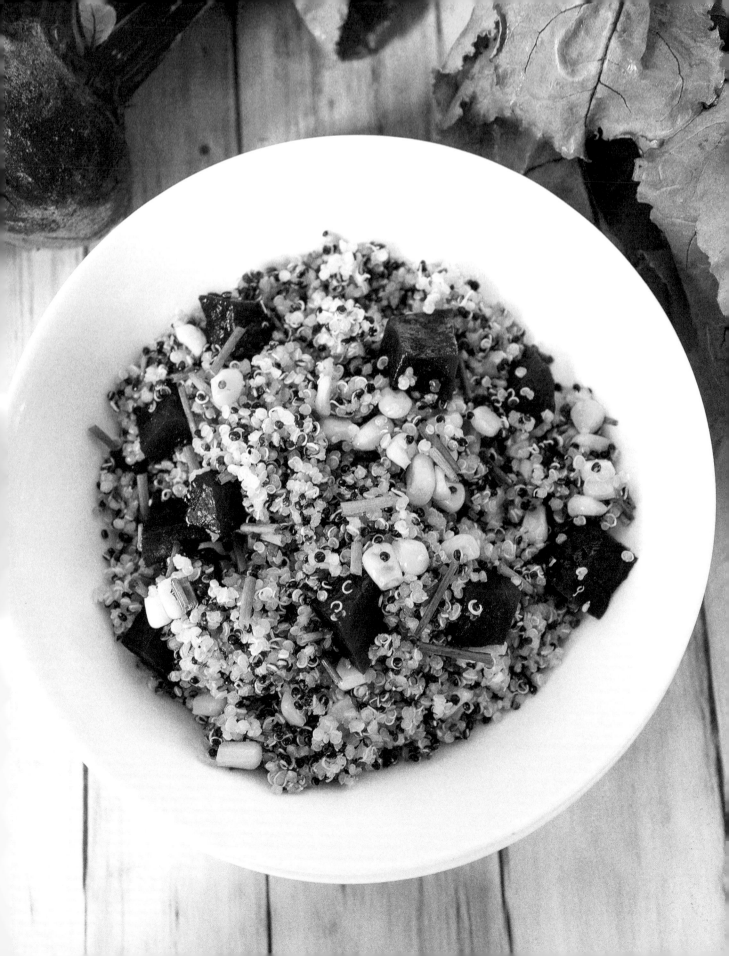

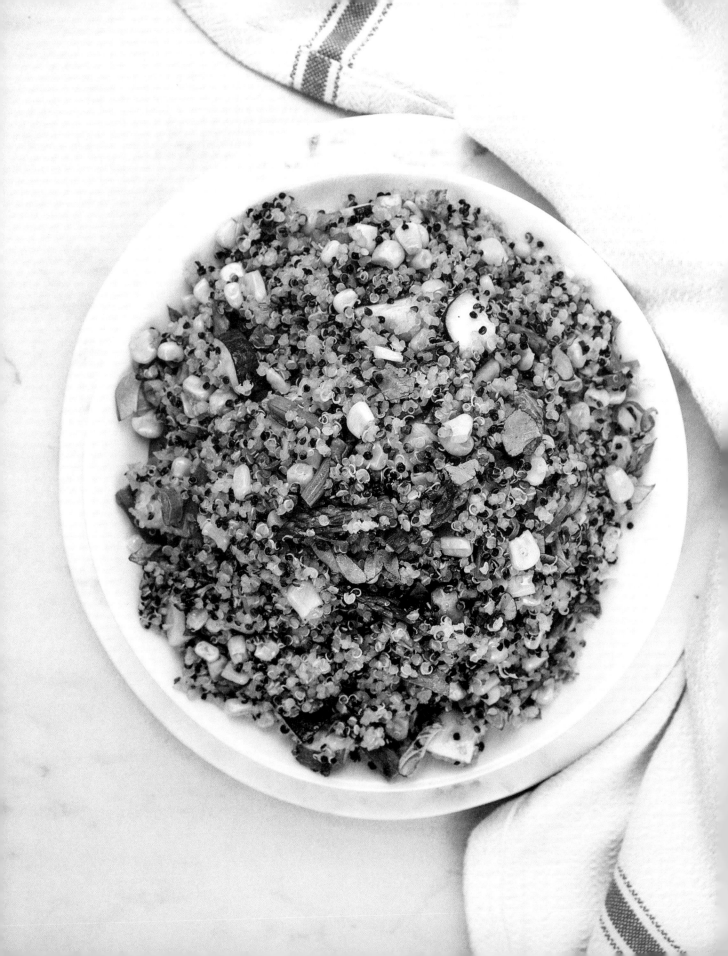

Summer Quinoa Salad

This quinoa salad boasts a complete plant protein with a summery twist. Zucchini and basil provide antioxidants and reduce inflammation, and of course olive oil is a healthy, anti-inflammatory fat.

····· CROWD PLEASER · HIGH PROTEIN · SUPERFOOD · VEGAN ·····

PREP TIME: 10 minutes • Cook Time: 20 minutes • Total Time: 30 minutes

1 cup dry tricolor quinoa

2 cups water

1 zucchini, diced

½ bunch asparagus

3 tablespoons extra-light olive oil, divided

2 ears corn on the cob or 2 cups frozen organic corn, thawed

2 tablespoons chopped garlic chives or scallions

½ cup chopped fresh basil

salt and pepper

1. Preheat the oven to 400°F.

2. In a pot over high heat, cook the quinoa in the water. When the water boils, reduce the heat to low and simmer for about 20 minutes or until all the liquid absorbs. Fluff with a fork and set aside.

3. Meanwhile, remove the woody ends of the asparagus and cut them into ½-inch pieces.

4. Toss the zucchini and asparagus with 1 tablespoon olive oil, spread on a baking sheet, and bake for 10 minutes.

5. Cut the kernels from the ears of corn or defrost the frozen corn.

6. In a bowl, combine the chives or scallions, basil, quinoa, zucchini, and corn. Add the remaining 2 tablespoons olive oil and salt and pepper to taste.

> **Variation**
>
> *Serve this dish warm or cold, depending on the season and your preference.*

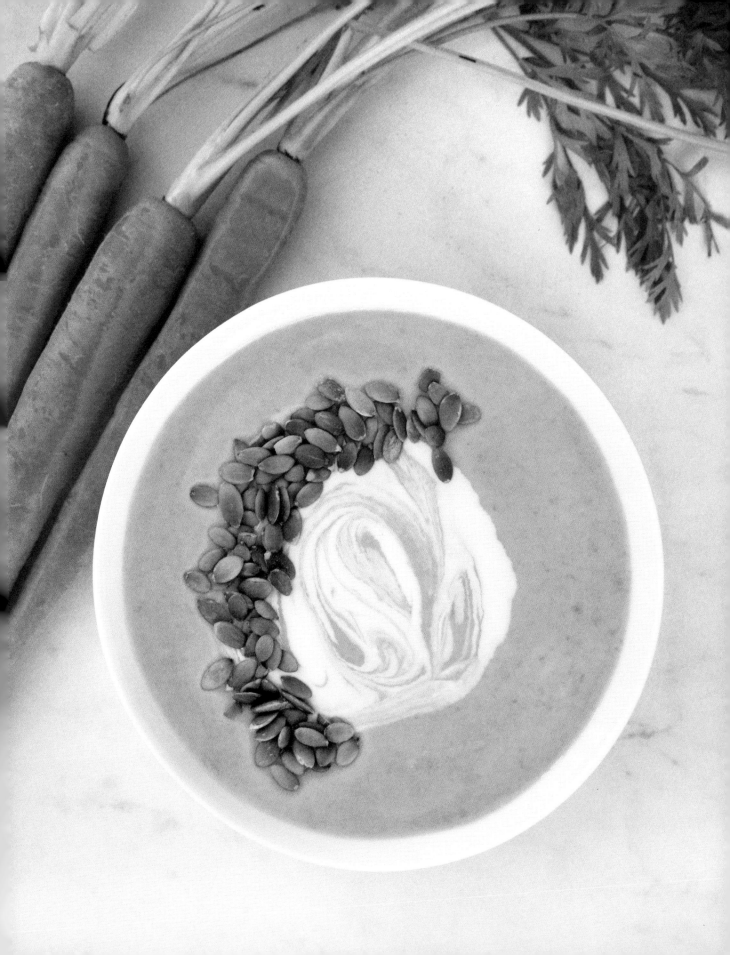

Acorn Squash Soup

This lovely soup comes together in a flash and is rich in vitamin A, fiber, quercetin, and other anti-inflammatory compounds from the ginger. The coconut cream adds a sweet background note, while the pumpkin seeds offer a little crunch to an otherwise smooth and creamy soup.

····· GREAT SNACK · LOW CAL · SUPERFOOD · VEGAN ·····

PREP TIME: 5 minutes · COOK TIME: 30 minutes · TOTAL TIME: 35 minutes

1 acorn squash

4 carrots

1 sweet onion

2 tablespoons olive oil

1 tablespoon grated ginger

1 teaspoon turmeric

1 cup water

1 (13½-ounce) can coconut
    cream, reserving
    2 tablespoons for garnish

¼ cup pumpkin seeds
    for garnish

1. Peel the squash, carrots, and onion and chop each into 1-inch cubes.

2. In a large saucepan over medium heat, add the olive oil, squash, carrots, and onions. Sauté for about 5–10 minutes until the vegetables start to brown, stirring every few minutes.

3. Add the ginger, turmeric, water, and coconut cream. Simmer over low heat for about 20 minutes, until the vegetables become tender.

4. Using an immersion blender, blend the soup until smooth and creamy.

5. Top with a drizzle of the reserved coconut cream and the pumpkin seeds.

> **Note**
>
> *Coconut cream has more coconut solids than coconut milk. When shopping for coconut cream, look for one without any stabilizing gums.*

Butternut Squash & Arugula Salad

Arugula, a peppery green, gives this salad a little kick. It's rich in antioxidants and vitamins A and C. To make this recipe even easier to make, roast extra squash and onions and freeze them in ½-cup portions. Then, when you're busy, you can just grab a portion to thaw.

····· GREAT SNACK · LOW CAL · SUPERFOOD · VEGAN ·····

PREP TIME: 10 minutes • COOK TIME: 25 minutes • TOTAL TIME: 35 minutes

1 small butternut squash

1 sweet onion

2 tablespoons olive oil

1 tablespoon maple syrup

1 pinch salt

8 cups arugula

1 apple, cored and diced, for garnish

DRESSING

4 tablespoons extra-virgin olive oil

2 tablespoons maple syrup

juice of ½ lemon

1 pinch salt

1. Preheat the oven to 400°F.

2. Dice the squash into ½-inch pieces and slice the onion.

3. Toss the squash and onion with the olive oil, maple syrup, and salt.

4. Place the vegetables on a baking sheet and roast them for 20–25 minutes or until they turn golden brown.

5. To make the dressing, in a small bowl, combine the extra-virgin olive oil, maple syrup, lemon juice, and salt.

6. Assemble the salad with arugula on the bottom and the squash and onions on top.

7. Drizzle the dressing over the salad and top with diced apples.

> ### Variation
>
> *For a crunchy twist to this recipe, use 1 cup freeze-dried apple chunks instead of fresh. Freeze-dried fruits dry so rapidly that they offer a great lower-histamine way to snack on fruit on the go. The fast-freeze method also locks in more nutrients and vitamin C. Also try watercress, another great nutrient-dense green, in this salad.*

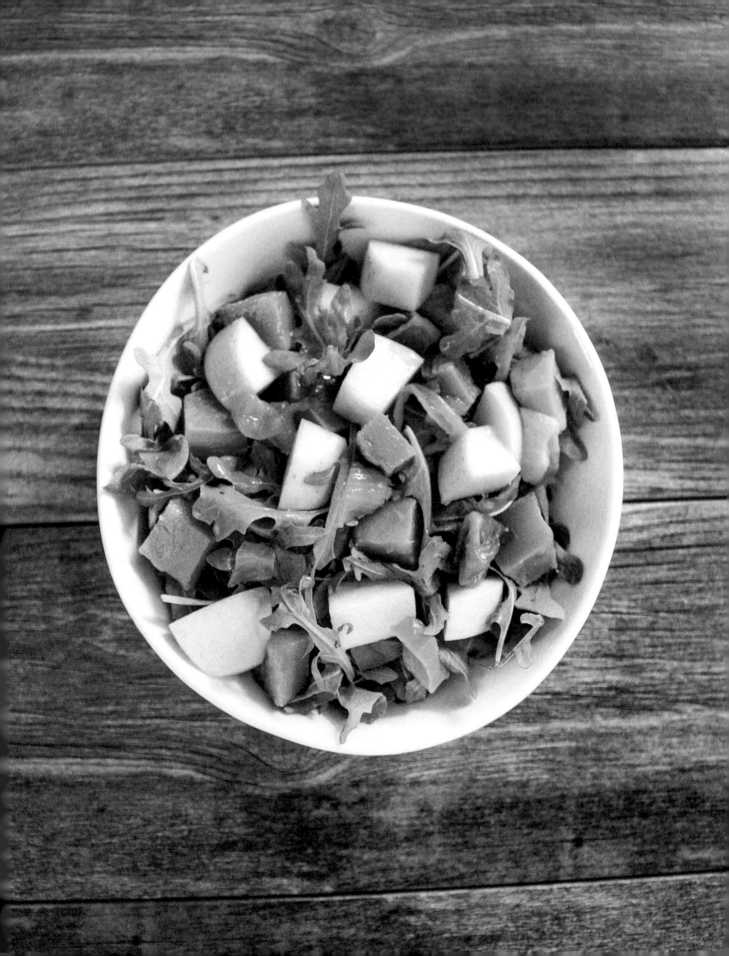

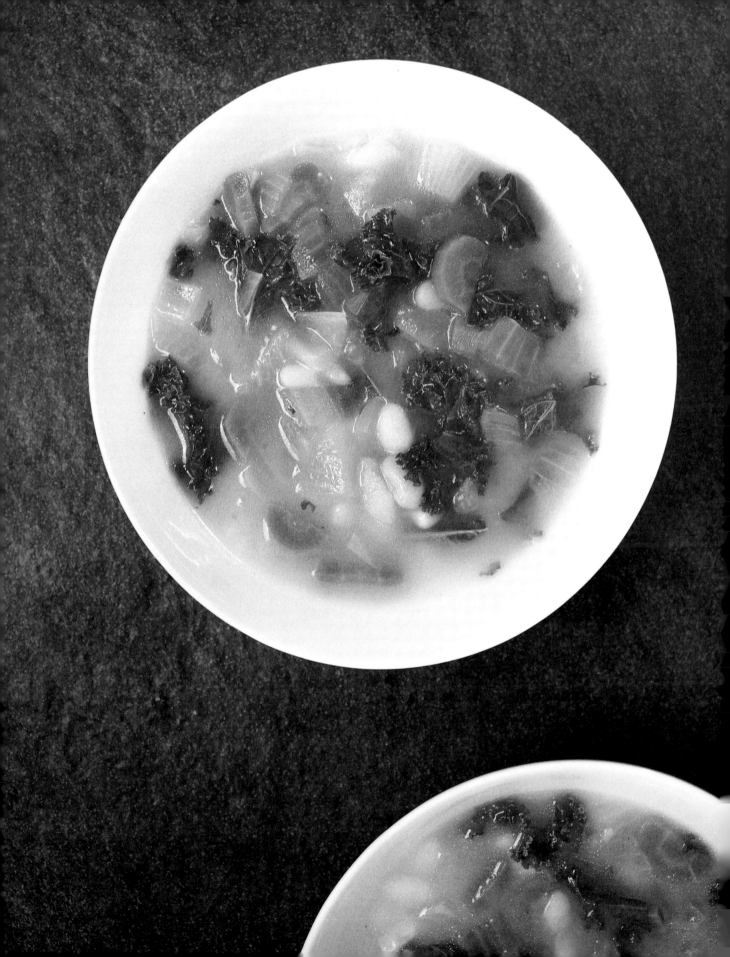

Kale & White Bean Soup

This delicate soup includes lots of vegetables rich in antioxidants, and the beans provide a nice plant-based protein. Avoid store-bought broths, though, which contain high levels of histamine, yeast, and additives that make them shelf-stable.

···· GREAT SNACK · SUPERFOOD · VEGAN ····

PREP TIME: 5 minutes • COOK TIME: 35 minutes • TOTAL TIME: 40 minutes

2 carrots

1 sweet onion

1 stalk celery

1 tablespoon extra-virgin olive oil

3 yellow potatoes, peeled and halved

4 cups Vegetable Broth (page 237) or water

½ teaspoon salt

2 bay leaves

1 teaspoon dried thyme or 1 tablespoon fresh thyme

½ bunch kale chopped, stems removed

2 cups white beans, cooked

1. Dice the carrots and onion and chop the celery.

2. In a medium pan over medium heat, sauté the carrots, onion, and celery in olive oil until tender, about 10 minutes.

3. Add the potatoes, broth or water, salt, bay leaves, and thyme. Simmer over medium-low heat for about 20 minutes or until the potatoes become tender.

4. Remove the potatoes with some broth and blend in food processor or blender. Add the potato mixture back to the pot to make a smooth, creamy soup.

5. Add the kale and beans and cook about 5 minutes or until the kale wilts and the beans warm.

6. Remove the bay leaves and discard.

Note
Freeze this soup in 2-cup portions for a quick lunch on a cold day.

Variation
You can use navy, cannellini, or great northern beans for this recipe.

Roasted Carrot & Garlic Hummus

You can eat this delicious dip as a snack or add it to a sandwich or wrap for a quick lunch. Freezing it in single portions makes this another prep-ahead, easy-grab lunch during a busy day. The sweetness of the carrots and roasted garlic play nicely with the creamy, white beans.

····· CROWD PLEASER · GREAT SNACK · HIGH PROTEIN · VEGAN ·····

PREP TIME: 20 minutes • COOK TIME: 20 minutes • TOTAL TIME: 40 minutes

2 carrots

1 clove garlic, skin on

1 cup cooked white beans
(cooked from dry or
defrosted)

2 tablespoons olive oil

1 teaspoon sesame seeds

2 tablespoons water

¼ teaspoon salt

1. Preheat oven to 400°F.

2. Peel and chop the carrots into 1-inch cubes.

3. Toss the carrots and garlic (skin on) in the olive oil. Spread them on a baking sheet and roast them for 15–20 minutes or until the carrots become tender and golden. Set aside.

4. In the bowl of a food processor, add the white beans, olive oil, sesame seeds, water, salt, and carrots.

5. Squeeze the garlic clove out of its skin, add it to the food processor, and puree until smooth. Add water to thin it out if necessary.

6. Serve with fresh vegetables or rice crackers or in a homemade wrap.

> **Tip**
>
> *Freeze the hummus in ice cube trays so you can take two cubes out for a proper portion.*
>
> **Variation**
>
> *You can use chickpeas or navy, cannellini, or great northern beans for this recipe.*

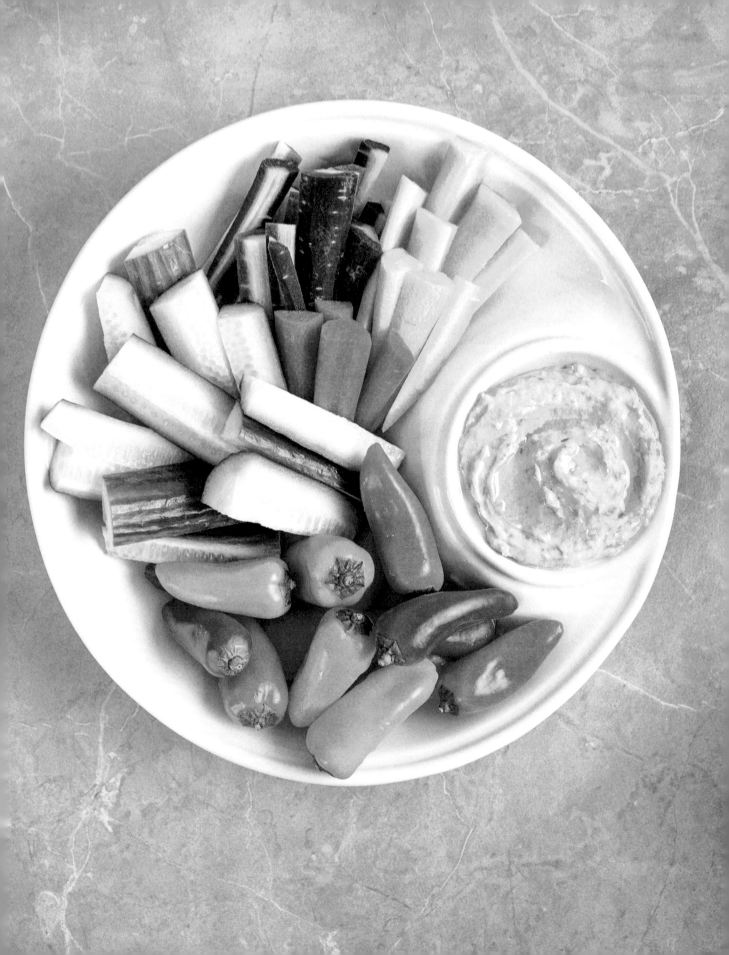

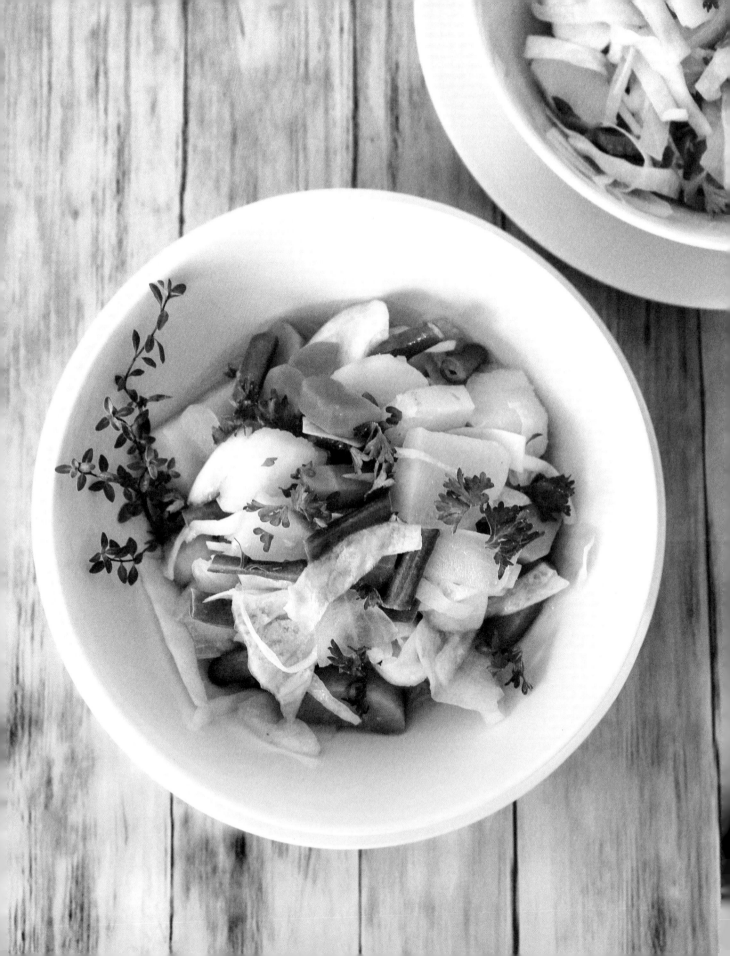

Superfood Stew

Cabbage—filled with liver-detoxifying compounds, anti-inflammatory agents, vitamin C, and fiber—is one of the most nutrient-dense vegetables available. This stew also features lots of thyme and parsley, which contain apigenin, a mast cell stabilizer.

····· LOW CAL · SUPERFOOD · VEGAN ·····

PREP TIME: 15 minutes • COOK TIME: 30 minutes • TOTAL TIME: 45 minutes

2 carrots

1 stalk celery

1 sweet onion

2 tablespoons extra-virgin olive oil

4 cups Vegetable Broth (page 237)

2 bay leaves

3 sprigs thyme, plus more for garnish

½ cup chopped fresh parsley, plus more for garnish

4 yellow potatoes, diced

1 teaspoon salt

1 small head green cabbage

2 cups chopped green beans

1. Dice the carrots, celery, and onion into mirepoix.

2. In a large pot, add the olive oil and mirepoix. Sauté over medium heat for about 10 minutes or until the vegetables cook all way through and become translucent.

3. Add the broth or water, bay leaves, thyme, parsley, potatoes, and salt and simmer over medium-low heat for another 10 minutes.

4. Add the cabbage and green beans and simmer over medium-low heat for 10 minutes or until the green vegetables are tender but still vibrant.

5. Remove the bay leaves and thyme stems, but keep the thyme leaves in the stew.

6. Garnish with fresh parsley and more thyme.

Note
Freeze this stew in single portions for making quick lunches.

Variation
To make this stew into a soup, simply add more broth or water to taste.

White Bean & Basil Cakes

These cakes are similar to veggie burgers, but they work better on a bed of lettuce than on buns. The basil and onion are anti-inflammatory, and beans are rich in prebiotic fiber for a healthy microbiome. If you make the caramelized onions ahead of time, freeze them, and thaw them, you can save some serious prep time on this recipe.

····· GREAT SNACK · HIGH PROTEIN · KID FRIENDLY · VEGAN ·····

PREP TIME: 10 minutes • COOK TIME: 1 hour • TOTAL TIME: 1 hour 10 minutes

2 large sweet onions

2 tablespoons water

5 tablespoons olive oil, divided

½ teaspoon salt

2 cups cooked white beans

½ cup rolled oats

1 clove garlic, minced, plus 1 clove for flavoring the sauté pan

¼ cup chopped fresh basil

1 cup crushed crispy rice cereal

1. Chop the onions.

2. In a medium pan over medium heat, combine the onions, water, 1 tablespoon olive oil, and salt. Cover, reduce heat to medium-low, and simmer for about 1 hour or until onions caramelize and become very tender.

3. In a large bowl, combine the white beans and oats and crush them together with a potato masher.

4. Add minced garlic, caramelized onions and basil to the bean mixture and stir to combine.

5. Preheat a skillet over medium heat and add 2 tablespoons olive oil and a clove of garlic.

6. Form the bean mixture into patties, dredge them in the crushed cereal, then sauté for about 4 minutes on each side or until golden and warmed through. Remove the clove of garlic before it gets too brown and bitter tasting.

7. Serve on a bed of greens.

Note

Try freezing these individually for a quick lunch. To reheat, place in the oven or toaster oven at 375°F for about 10–15 minutes.

Tip

These bean cakes also work great as vegan "meatballs" over gluten-free pasta. They go particularly well with Zucchini Noodles (page 159) and Vegan Pesto (page 236).

Variation

You can use navy, cannellini, or great northern beans for this recipe.

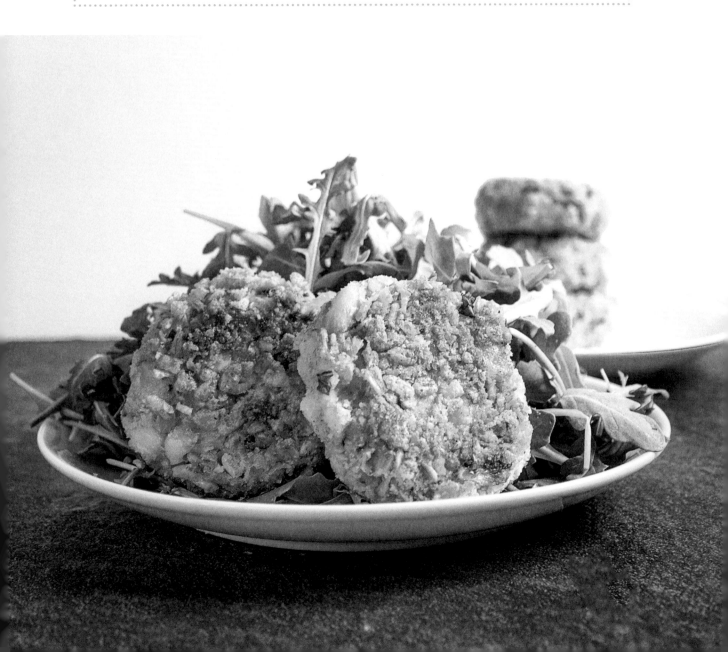

SIDES

Garlic Broccoli

This versatile veggie dish has lots of vitamin C to boost DAO enzyme production as well as having detoxifying phytochemicals. It's a bright burst of nutrition and also sweet and savory. A little coconut sugar or brown sugar sweetens the deal and makes it more of a treat.

····· FAST · LOW CAL · SUPERFOOD · VEGAN ·····

PREP TIME: 3 minutes • COOK TIME: 12 minutes • TOTAL TIME: 15 minutes

2 heads broccoli

1 red bell pepper

1 clove garlic

1 white onion

salt

1 tablespoon extra-light olive oil or sesame oil

¼ cup water

2 tablespoons coconut or brown sugar

1. Chop the broccoli, slice the bell pepper, and mince the garlic.

2. Slice the onion last to prevent kitchen tears.

3. In a medium pan over medium heat, add the vegetables, salt to taste, and oil.

4. Add the water to help the vegetables cook.

5. Sauté for about 10 minutes or until the vegetables become tender.

6. Add the sugar and stir for 1–2 minutes.

Tip

This dish pairs well with the Ginger Vegetable Fried Rice with Sautéed Bok Choy (page 188 or Sesame Chicken (page 194). Add it to a serving of brown rice or quinoa to make a quick vegan meal.

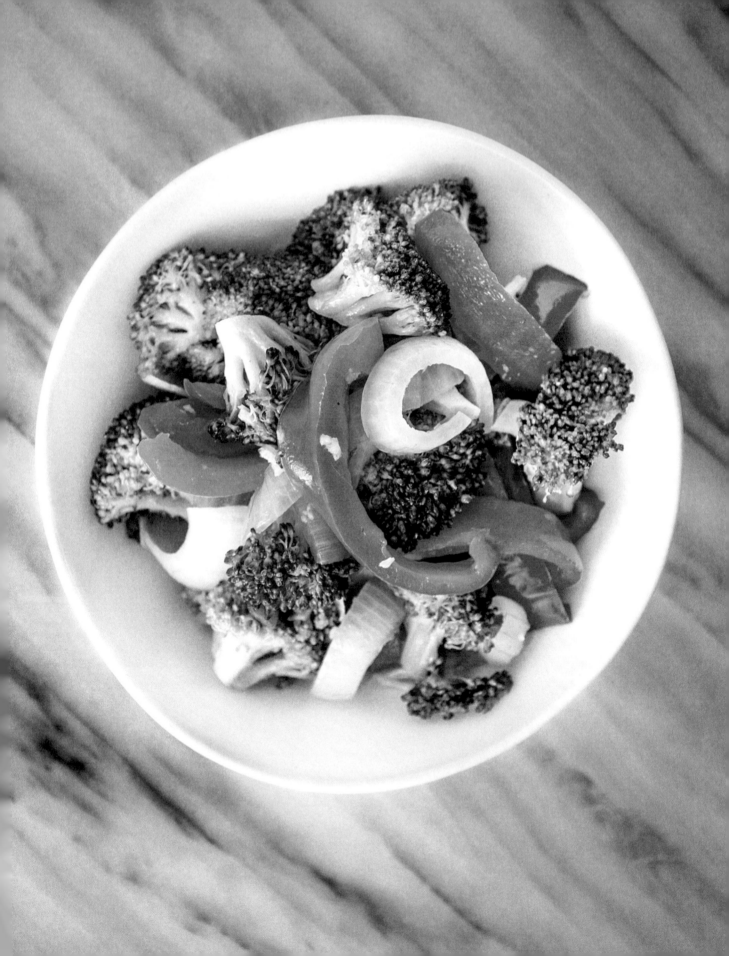

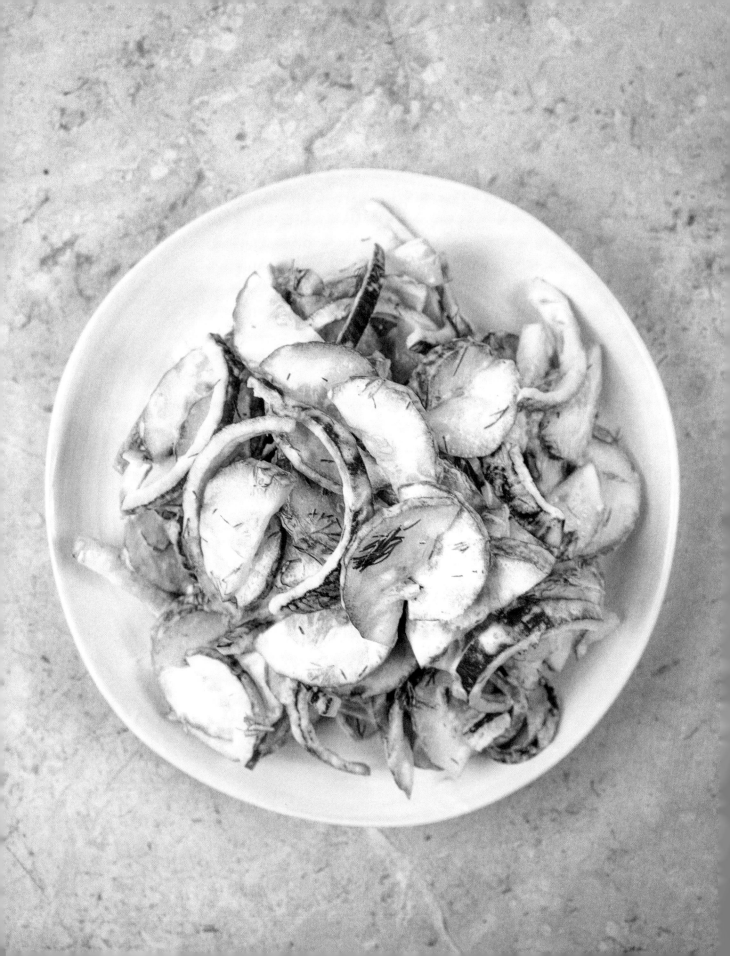

Cucumber Dill Salad

This cucumber salad is simple and delicious and makes a great dish at a summer barbecue or cookout. Mascarpone cheese is a great way to make a creamy low-histamine dressing blended with fresh herbs.

····· FAST · LOW CAL · VEGETARIAN ·····

PREP TIME: 15 minutes • TOTAL TIME: 15 minutes

1 large European cucumber

½ red onion

¼ cup chopped fresh dill, plus 2 tablespoons for garnish

2 tablespoons chopped fresh chives

¼ cup mascarpone cheese

2 tablespoons extra-light olive oil

½ teaspoon salt

1. Slice the cucumber into ¼-inch half rounds, and slice the red onion as well.

2. In a large bowl, combine the cucumber and onions.

3. In a food processor or blender, add the dill, chives, mascarpone, olive oil, and salt and pulse until just combined and smooth.

4. Add the dill mixture to the cucumbers and onions, stir to combine thoroughly, and garnish with more dill.

5. Let sit for 5–10 minutes before serving to marinate the flavors.

Tip

Serve this cucumber salad with the Grilled Chicken & Vegetables (page 156) or Black Bean Burgers.

Variation

To make this salad vegan, omit the mascarpone cheese from step 3 and blend together the herbs, oil, and salt, along with a squeeze of lemon juice.

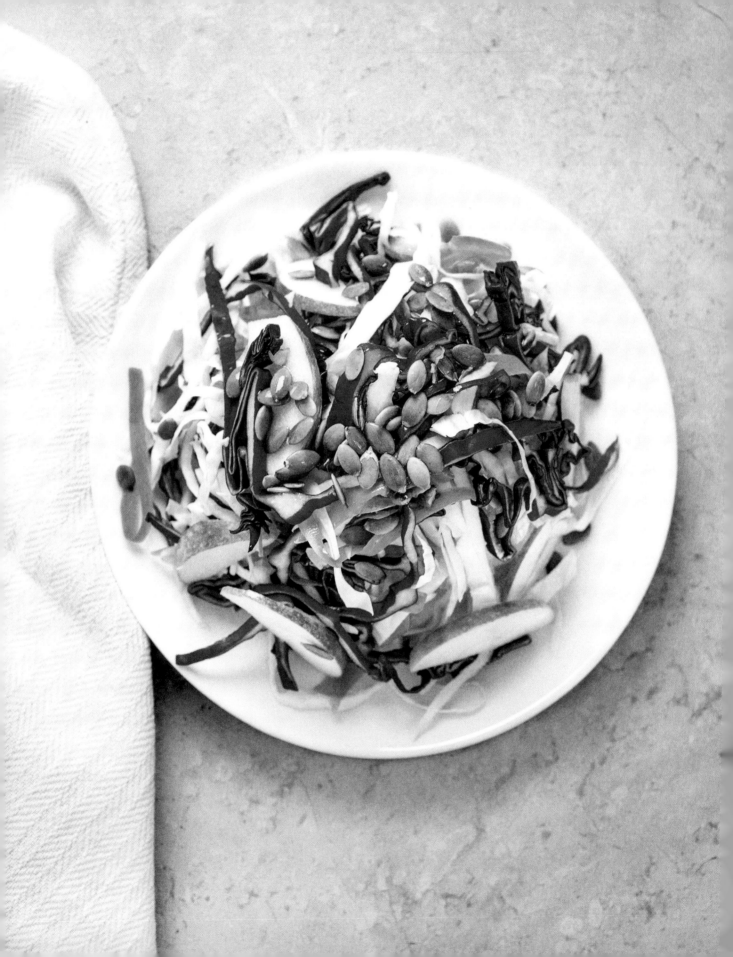

Fall Harvest Salad

This quick-and-easy salad contains lots of cabbage, which boasts high levels of vitamin C, anti-inflammatories, and liver detoxifiers. It has a lot of crunch to it and works nicely as a side to any meal or as a serve-alone lunch option.

····· FAST · LOW CAL · SUPERFOOD · VEGAN ·····

PREP TIME: 15 minutes • TOTAL TIME: 15 minutes

1 carrot

1 red apple

2 cups thinly sliced red cabbage

1 cup thinly sliced green cabbage

juice of ½ lemon, divided

1 tablespoon maple syrup

1 pinch salt

2 tablespoons extra-virgin olive oil

¼ cup raw pumpkin seeds

1. Thinly shred the carrot with a vegetable peeler.

2. Thinly slice the apple and brush it with a little lemon juice to prevent browning.

3. In a medium bowl, combine the cabbages, carrot, and apple.

4. In a small bowl, combine the lemon juice, maple syrup, salt, and olive oil. Stir to combine thoroughly.

5. Toss the dressing with the vegetables and top with the pumpkin seeds.

Tip

This is a great winter salad. It holds up well so you won't have any wilt if it sits on a holiday table for a little while. It also works nicely as a base for a dinner with roasted or grilled salmon.

Variation

Use different fruits, such as sliced grapes instead of the apples, for a slightly different variation.

Summer Succotash

Succotash is a delicious mix of corn and fresh shelling beans. If you can't find shelling beans, use black beans instead. Fresh summer sweet corn lifts the heaviness of the beans, and it adds just a hint of a crunch. Swiss chard boosts the nutrition and anti-inflammatory power of this dish, which also makes a great stand-alone lunch. Make this recipe for your next cookout or picnic.

····· CROWD PLEASER · SUPERFOOD · VEGAN ·····

PREP TIME: 10 minutes · COOK TIME: 10 minutes · TOTAL TIME: 20 minutes

3 scallions

2 tablespoons butter or extra-light olive oil

2 cups chopped Swiss chard

4 cups organic sweet corn, fresh or thawed from frozen

1 cup black beans, cooked from dry or thawed from frozen, or shelling beans

salt and pepper

1. Chop the scallions.

2. In a large saucepan, add the butter or olive oil, scallions, Swiss chard, and corn. Sauté until tender, about 8 minutes.

3. Add the cooked beans and sauté for 2–3 more minutes, until the beans have warmed.

4. Season with salt and pepper to taste.

> **Note**
>
> *Similar to dried beans, shelling beans are available at the end of the summer harvest. Typically they're sold fresh at the end of the summer and then dried and sold throughout the year. Butter beans, cannellini beans, and cranberry beans are all easily available shelling beans.*

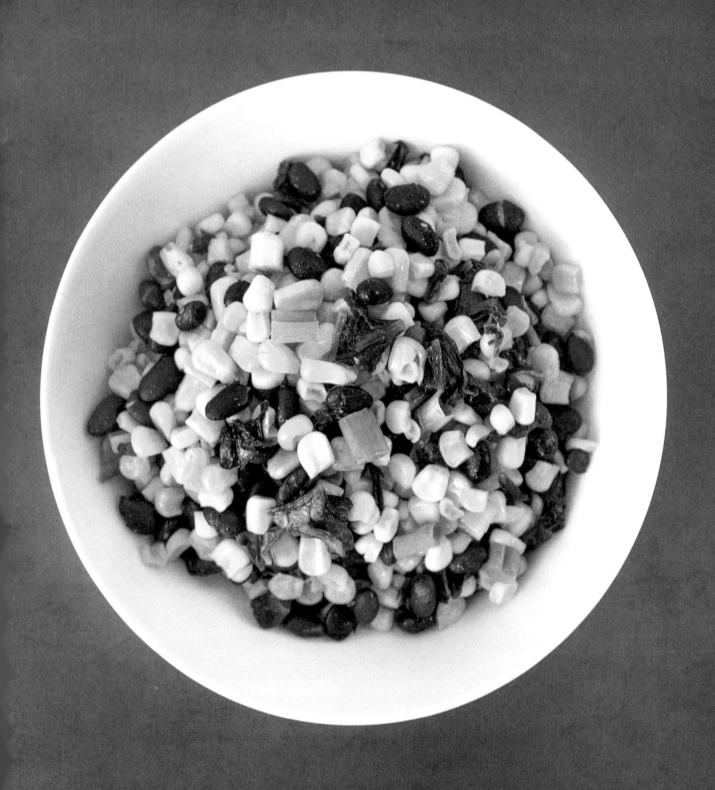

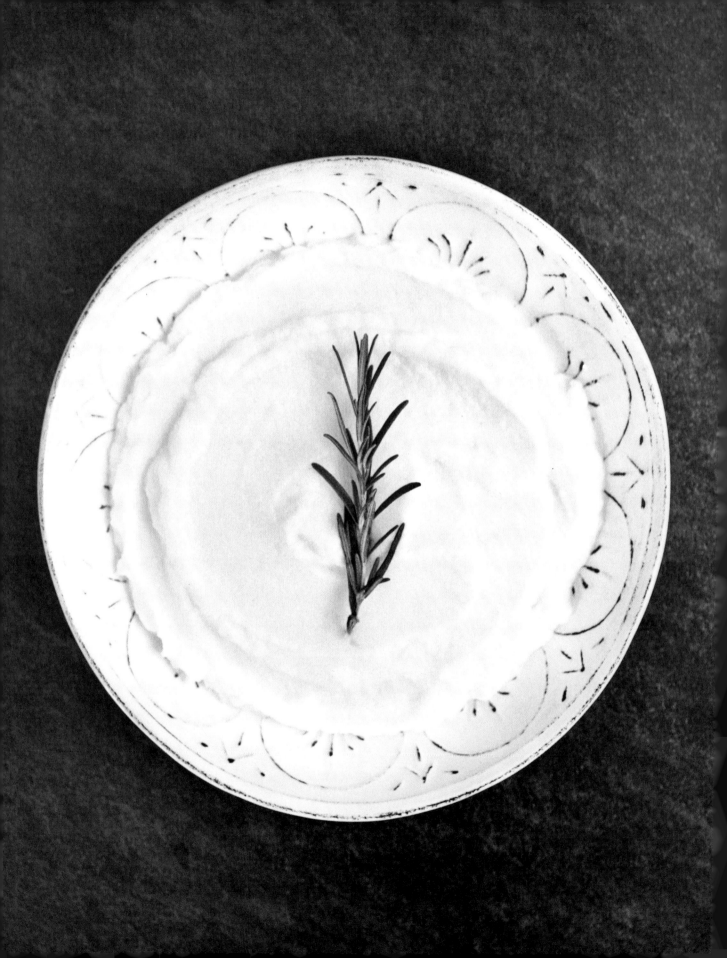

Cauliflower Mash

Do you love mashed potatoes but want more nutrition and fewer carbs? Try this dish. Rich in sulfur compounds, cauliflower is an excellent detoxifier. Steaming it helps to retain more nutrients than boiling, and the garlic adds just a hint of zing to liven it up.

····· CROWD PLEASER · KID FRIENDLY · LOW CAL · SUPERFOOD · VEGETARIAN ·····

PREP TIME: 10 minutes · COOK TIME: 15 minutes · TOTAL TIME: 25 minutes

1 head cauliflower
1 clove garlic
¼ cup milk or Vegetable Broth (page 237)
2 tablespoons butter
1 pinch salt

1. Chop the head of cauliflower.

2. In a large pot filled with an inch of water, add the cauliflower to a steamer basket along with the garlic. Cover and steam for 10–15 minutes or until tender.

3. Add the steamed cauliflower and garlic to the bowl of your food processor. Add milk or broth and the butter and salt. Puree until smooth.

Note

Have this side dish with the Oven-Fried Chicken (page 183) or Beef Tenderloin with Herb Butter (page 196).

Variation

Thin this recipe with more milk and broth and use it as a sauce for pasta. It easily becomes a skinny version of a cheeseless alfredo.

Make your next batch of mashed potatoes with half the carbs but more nutrition by using half of this recipe to substitute for half of the potatoes.

Maple Thyme Carrots

Carrots are a naturally rich source of beta-carotene, a powerful antioxidant. These carrots, however, taste like little candy morsels. With these around, you won't have any problem wanting to eat healthy. The thyme balances the sweetness and provides antihistamine and anti-inflammatory properties.

····· CROWD PLEASER · GREAT SNACK · KID FRIENDLY · VEGAN ·····

PREP TIME: **5 minutes** • COOK TIME: **30 minutes** • TOTAL TIME: **35 minutes**

6 carrots

1 tablespoon maple syrup

1 teaspoon extra-virgin
   olive oil

1 teaspoon chopped fresh
   thyme

1 pinch salt

1. Preheat the oven to 375°F.

2. Peel the carrots and cut them in half lengthwise.

3. Toss the carrots in the maple syrup, olive oil, thyme, and salt. Use your hands to coat them evenly.

4. Spread the carrots on a baking sheet and roast for 15 minutes.

5. Flip them over and roast for another 15 minutes, until they turn golden brown and start to caramelize.

Note

Carrots come in many different colors, and each color provides different antioxidants. Purple carrots look interesting and provide the carotenoid compounds in orange carrots while also adding anthocyanin. Most grocery stores carry a variety of colors, or you can grow different colors in your kitchen garden.

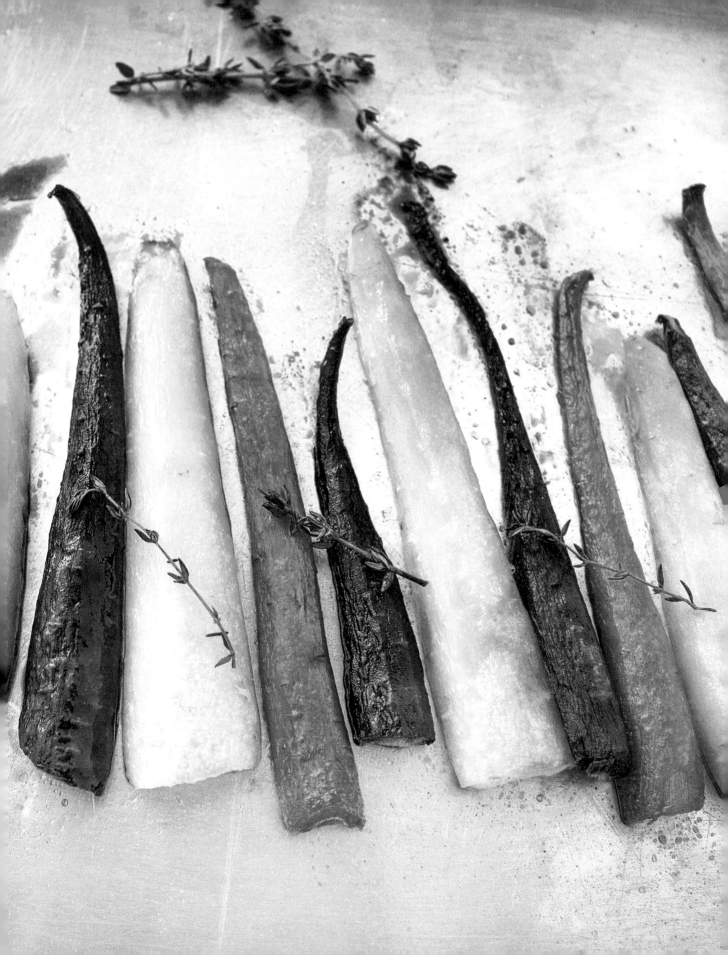

Rosemary Sea Salt Brussels Sprouts

Brussels sprouts have a bad reputation, but that's because so many people grew up eating them the wrong way. Boiling them to death destroys most of their nutrients—lots of vitamins A and C. Roasting them, on the other hand, keeps them nice and crispy, enhances their natural taste (rather than transforming it into something weird), and gives them a nice, golden sheen. Rosemary is a great source of rosmarinic acid, a natural antihistamine.

····· GREAT SNACK · LOW CAL · SUPERFOOD · VEGAN ·····

PREP TIME: **10 minutes** • COOK TIME: **25 minutes** • TOTAL TIME: **35 minutes**

1 pound Brussels sprouts

2 tablespoons chopped fresh rosemary

2 tablespoons extra-virgin olive oil

½ teaspoon sea salt

1. Preheat the oven to 400°F.

2. Remove the stems from the sprouts and halve the Brusells sprouts lengthwise.

3. In a bowl, combine the Brussels sprouts, rosemary, olive oil, and sea salt. Use your hands to mix them together, coating well.

4. Peel the Brussels sprouts apart so the outer layers get extra crispy.

5. Spread the sprouts evenly on a baking sheet and roast for 20–25 minutes, until they turn golden brown.

Note

Serve this dish at your next holiday meal. The Brussels sprouts pair well with the Rosemary & Garlic Chicken Breasts with Vegetables (page 200).

Variation

Make these with a drizzle of maple syrup, olive oil, and salt. They taste sweet and crispy, like veggie candy, which will appeal to picky young palates.

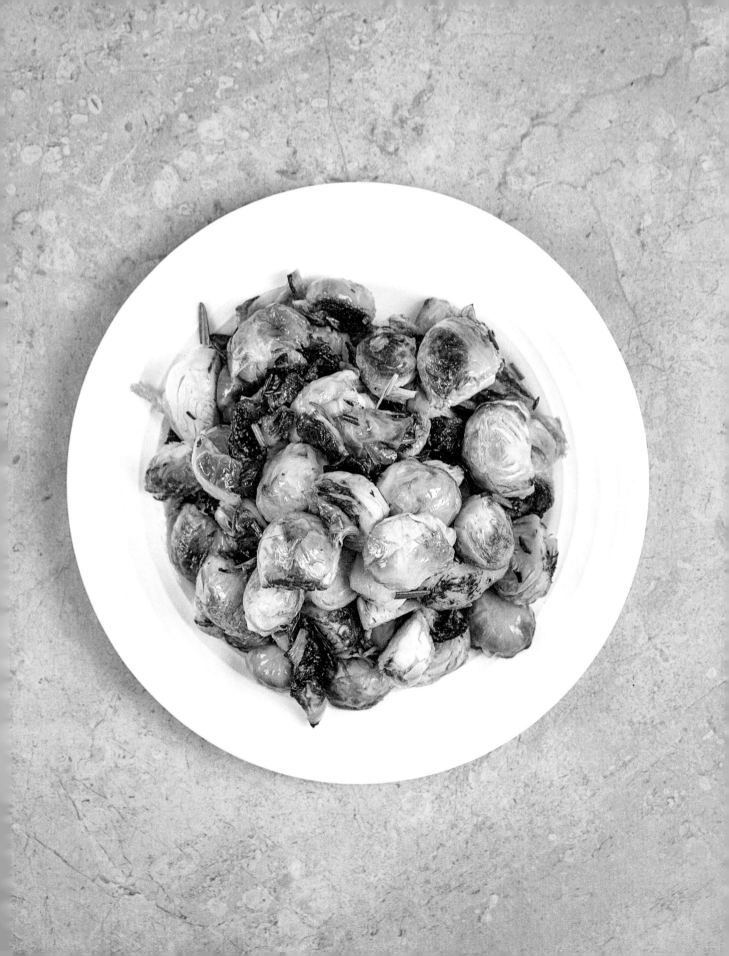

Roasted Vegetables

This dazzling array of vegetables makes for a great side dish that's bursting with flavonoids, carotenoids, and antioxidants. In the winter, you can use these as a salad base instead of lettuce, or you can go one better and serve them on a bed of greens or cooked kale for even more anti-inflammatory goodness. Roast up a large pan on the weekend and batch portions for a quick way to round out a meal.

····· CROWD PLEASER · LOW CAL · VEGAN ·····

PREP TIME: **20** minutes • COOK TIME: **20** minutes • TOTAL TIME: **40** minutes

5 carrots

3 beets

1 large sweet potato

1 purple sweet potato or
     purple potato

1 large sweet or purple onion

3 tablespoons extra-light
     olive oil

1 pinch salt

1. Preheat the oven to 400°F.

2. Peel and cut the carrots and beets into ½-inch to 1-inch chunks.

3. Cut the sweet potatoes into ½-inch to 1-inch chunks.

4. Peel and cut the onion into ½-inch to 1-inch chunks. (Cut the onion last to avoid kitchen tears.)

5. Toss the vegetables with the olive oil and salt.

6. Spread them evenly on a baking sheet and roast them for 10 minutes.

7. Flip them carefully with a spatula and roast for another 10 minutes.

> **Tip**
>
> *Freeze the veggies in airtight single-serving containers or resealable freezer bags for up to 3 months.*

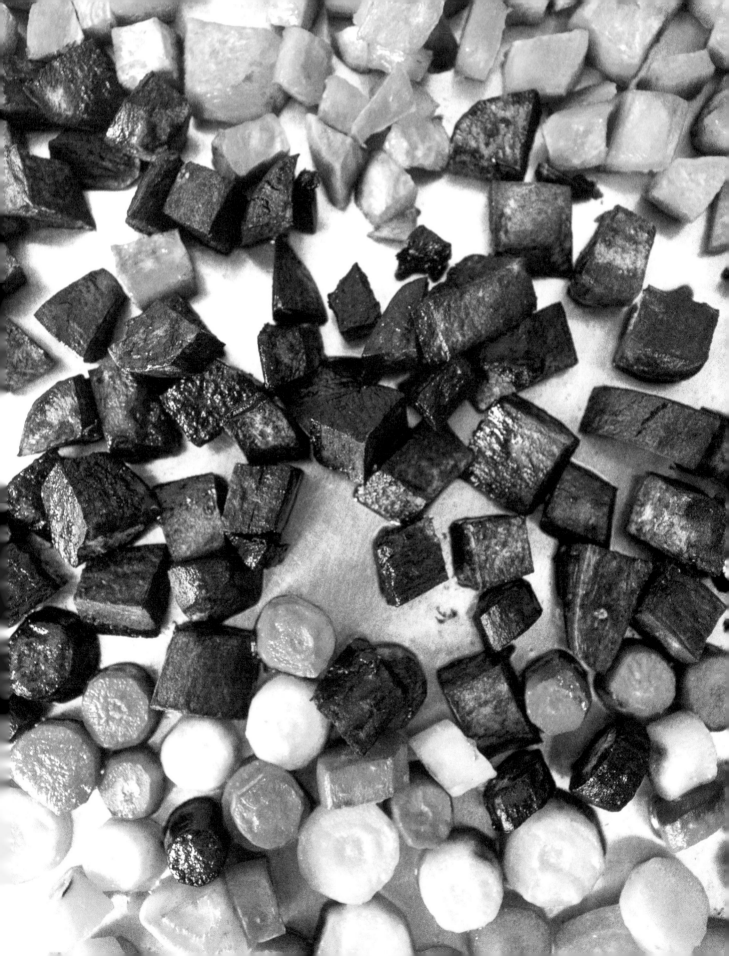

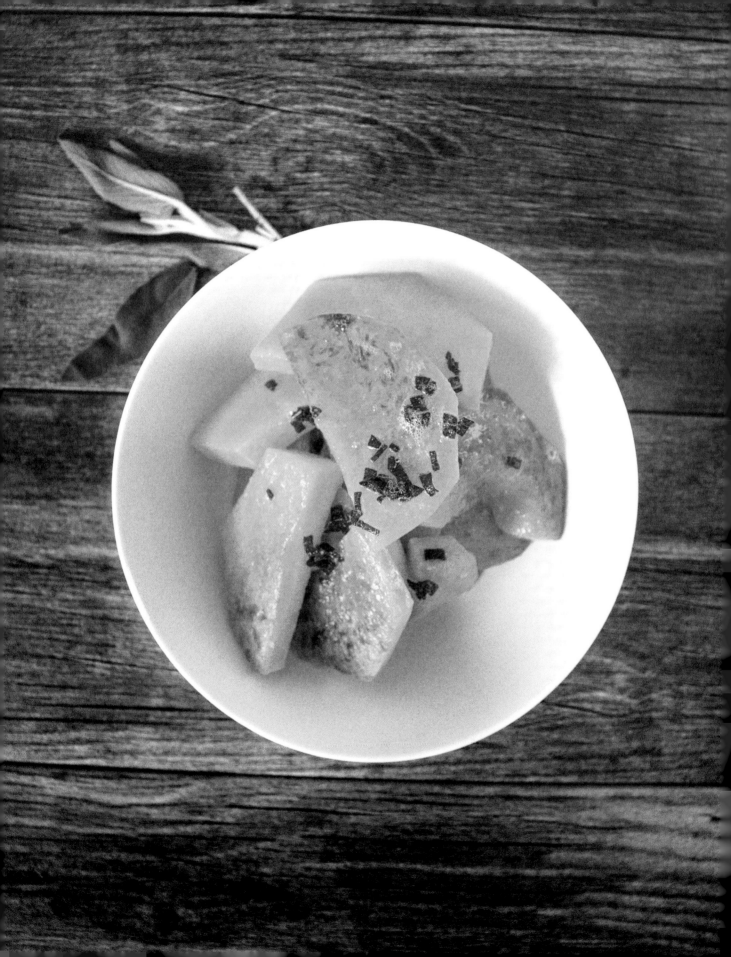

Butternut Squash with Brown Butter & Sage

This simple squash recipe will remind you instantly of fall and specifically Thanksgiving. The butter boosts the taste of the whole dish and highlights the natural sweetness of the roasted squash. The sage provides a nice herbal balance.

····· CROWD PLEASER · GREAT SNACK · SUPERFOOD · VEGETARIAN ·····

PREP TIME: 10 minutes • COOK TIME: 35 minutes • TOTAL TIME: 45 minutes

1 large butternut squash

1 tablespoon extra-virgin olive oil

¼ cup butter

4 sage leaves, chopped

½ teaspoon salt

1. Preheat the oven to 400°F.

2. Peel the squash, remove the seeds, and chop it into ½-inch chunks.

3. Coat the squash chunks in the olive oil and spread them on a baking sheet.

4. Roast them for about 30 minutes or until the squash turns golden brown. Remove them from the oven and set aside.

5. In a large skillet over medium heat, add the butter and sage leaves and cook them for about 5 minutes or until the butter starts to brown.

6. Toss the butternut squash with the browned sage butter and top with a sprinkle of salt.

> **Tip**
>
> *Toss the squash with gluten-free pasta or gnocchi. It also makes a great filling for a savory crepe or served over greens with roasted chicken or salmon.*

Onion Rings

Yes, healthy onion rings! Onions provide rich amounts of quercetin, which just goes to show that you can have an indulgent recipe that's low-histamine! Everyone craves fried food once in a while, and this side will satisfy that urge with healthy fats, fewer calories, and anti-inflammatory ingredients. Dredging the onions might seem a little time-consuming, but it's well worth the effort.

····· CROWD PLEASER · DAIRY FREE · GREAT SNACK · KID FRIENDLY ·····
LOW CAL · VEGETARIAN

PREP TIME: 30 minutes • COOK TIME: 20 minutes • TOTAL TIME: 50 minutes

4 tablespoons extra-light olive oil, divided
3 tablespoons All-Purpose Flour Blend (page 28)
½ teaspoon baking powder
½ teaspoon paprika
½ teaspoon salt, plus more to taste
1 large or 2 small sweet onions
1 egg, beaten
1 cup crushed crispy rice cereal

1. Preheat the oven to 400°F.

2. Line a baking sheet with aluminum foil and drizzle with 2 tablespoons of olive oil.

3. On a plate or in a bowl, mix the All-Purpose Flour Blend, baking powder, paprika, and salt.

4. Slice the onions into ⅓-inch rings.

5. Dredge the rings in the flour mixture and set aside.

6. Set up two shallow dishes, one containing the beaten egg, the other with the crushed cereal.

7. One at a time, dip the flour-coated onions in the egg, then the rice cereal, and place them on the prepared baking sheet.

8. Drizzle the onions with the remaining 2 tablespoons of olive oil and season with a pinch of salt.

9. Bake the onion rings for 10 minutes on one side, then flip them and bake for 10 more minutes on the other side or until they are crispy and brown.

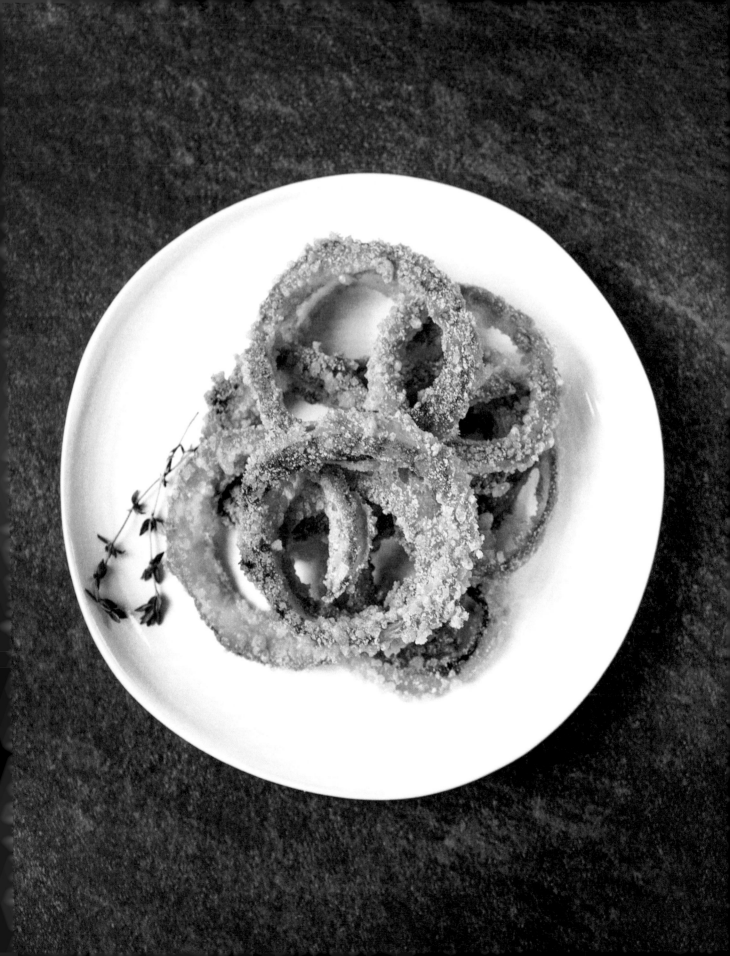

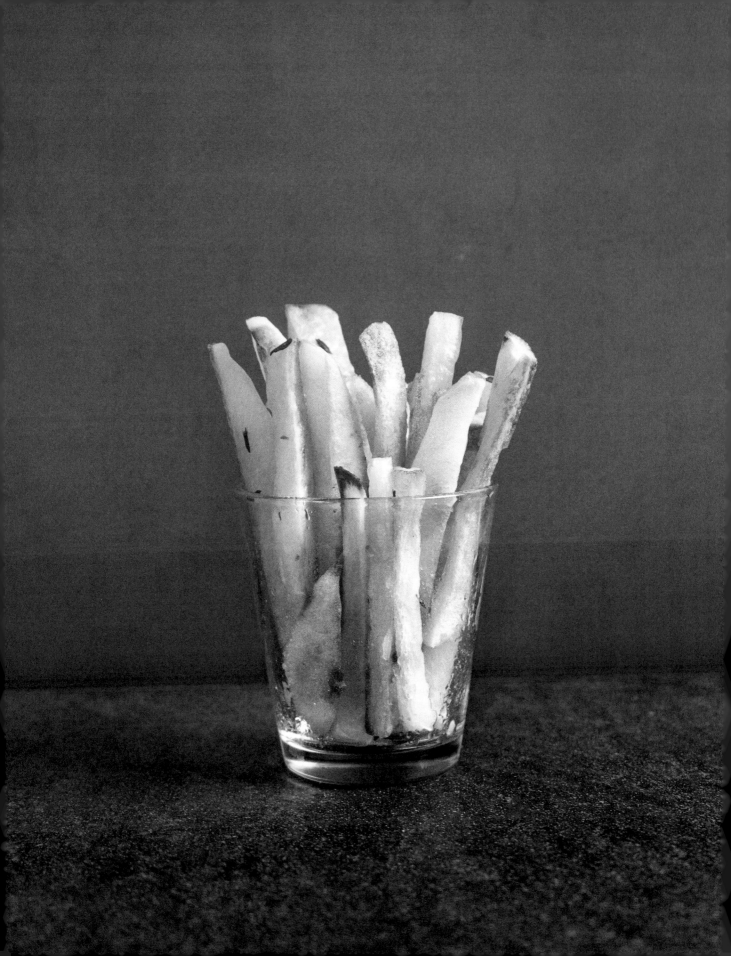

Thyme Garlic Fries

Who doesn't love fries? The two keys to this recipe are the olive oil and a long cooking time to increase the crispiness without drowning the potatoes in excess fat. You can use regular potatoes or sweet potatoes in this recipe. Tossing them with garlic and thyme makes them taste even better, and it also increases the dish's histamine-lowering properties.

····· CROWD PLEASER · GREAT SNACK · KID FRIENDLY · VEGAN ·····
PREP TIME: 15 minutes • COOK TIME: 45 minutes • TOTAL TIME: 1 hour

6 yellow potatoes or
    2 large sweet potatoes
1 clove garlic
2 tablespoons extra-light
    olive oil
2 tablespoons chopped fresh
    thyme
½ teaspoon sea salt

1. Preheat the oven to 400°F.

2. Slice the potatoes into ¼-inch sticks and mince the garlic.

3. Toss the fries with the garlic, olive oil, thyme, and salt, using your hands to coat evenly.

4. Spread the fries on a baking sheet and bake for 30 minutes, until the bottoms turn golden.

5. Using a spatula, carefully flip the fries. Bake for an additional 15 minutes on the other side until crispy and golden.

Variation

Use purple potatoes. They have incredible health benefits and a slightly different flavor profile, but they still taste like a treat. If you can't find them at your grocery store, check out your local farmers' market for a good selection.

DINNER

Mango Salsa Salmon

Mango salsa gives the tender salmon in this recipe a zip of color, flavor, and a boost of vitamin C to help with decreasing histamine levels. The omega-3 fatty acids in the salmon also help reduce inflammation.

····· DAIRY FREE · HIGH PROTEIN ·····

PREP TIME: 5 minutes • COOK TIME: 15 minutes • TOTAL TIME: 20 minutes

1 pound salmon, cut into
    4 portions
2 tablespoons olive oil,
    divided
1 pinch salt
2 bunches fresh asparagus
2 teaspoons olive oil, divided
Mango Salsa (page 230)

1. Preheat the oven to 400°F.

2. Drizzle a baking sheet with 1 tablespoon olive oil and place the salmon portions on it, adding a pinch of salt to the salmon.

3. Bake for 15 minutes or until the salmon flesh flakes lightly with fork.

4. Meanwhile, remove the tough ends of the asparagus and discard, then toss the spears with 1 tablespoon olive oil.

5. On a baking sheet, bake the asparagus for 10 minutes or until it starts to brown.

6. While the salmon is baking, prepare the Mango Salsa.

7. When the salmon has finished cooking, top it with Mango Salsa and serve with the roasted asparagus.

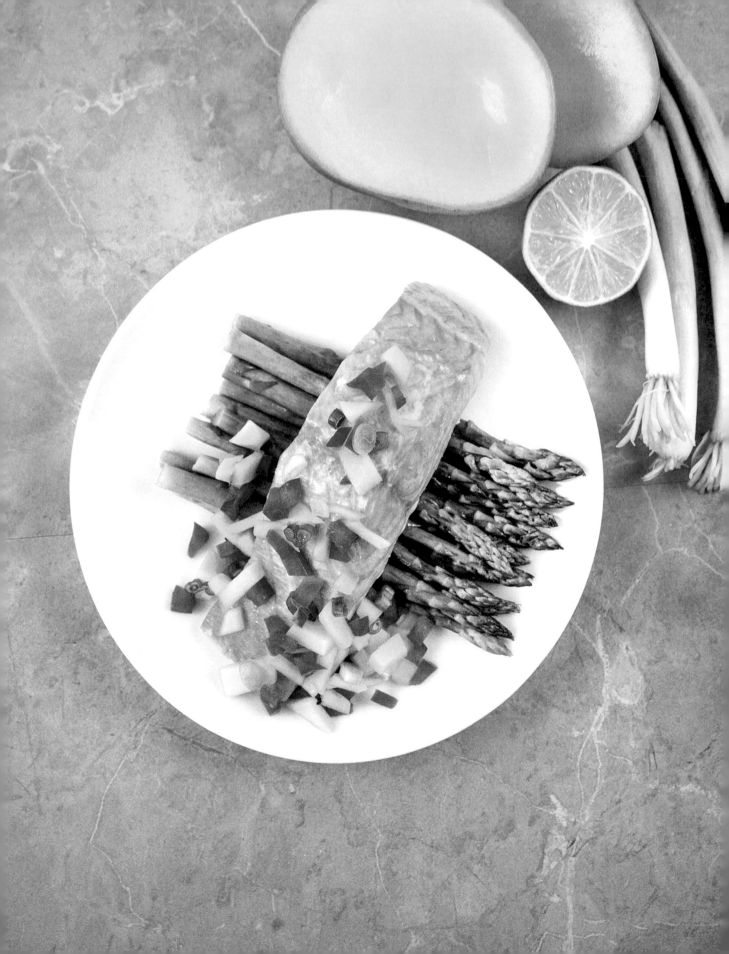

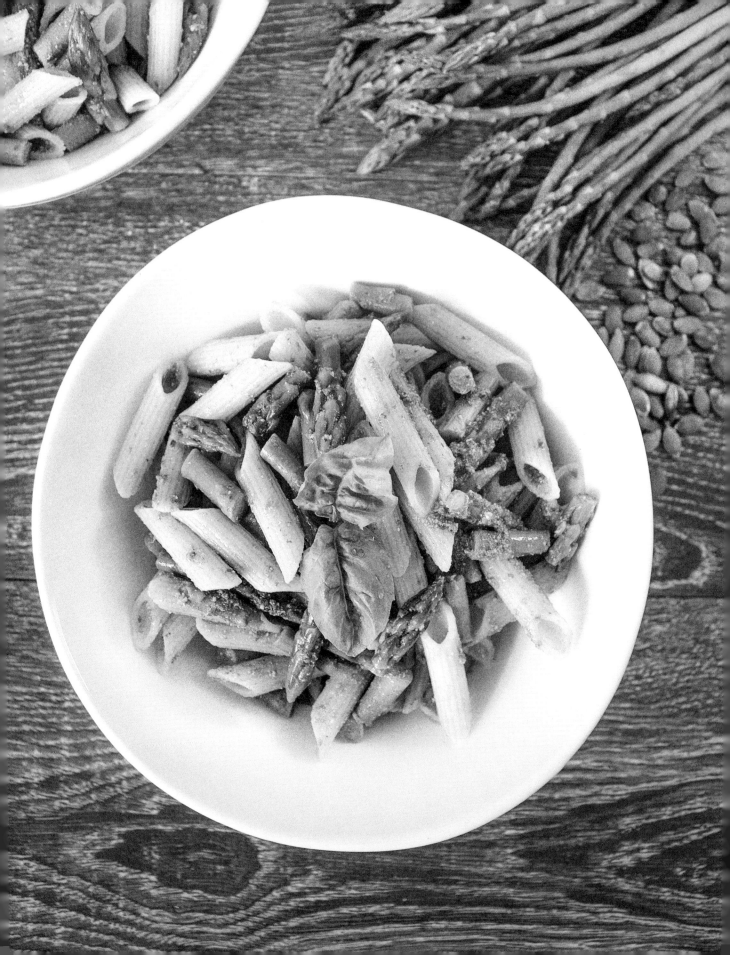

Pesto Penne with Asparagus

Pesto is a great option for low-histamine pasta dressing without using tomatoes. It's rich in basil flavonoids, olive oil, and pumpkin seeds, but sunflower seeds would work well too. Adding a hint of lemon brightens up the pesto and keeps it from turning brown. Swiss chard adds even more greens and nutrients to the dish.

····· CROWD PLEASER · KID FRIENDLY · VEGAN ·····

PREP TIME: 5 minutes • COOK TIME: 15 minutes • TOTAL TIME: 20 minutes

1 (12-ounce) package gluten-free noodles

Vegan Pesto (page 236)

1 bunch asparagus

1 teaspoon extra-virgin olive oil

basil for garnish

1. Cook the pasta according to package instructions. Rinse under hot water to remove remaining starch.

2. Meanwhile, prepare the Vegan Pesto. Add a little extra olive oil to thin the pesto if needed.

3. Remove the tough, woody ends from the asparagus and discard. Slice the stalks into ½-inch pieces.

4. In a medium skillet over medium heat, sauté the asparagus chunks in the olive oil for about 5 minutes or until the asparagus starts to brown and become tender-crisp.

5. Toss the pasta, pesto, and asparagus together, stirring thoroughly to distribute the pesto evenly.

6. Garnish with fresh basil.

Note

Gluten-free pasta sticks together more than wheat-based pastas. Add a little olive oil to the cooking water to help prevent sticking, rinse with hot water to remove excess starch, and then add a little more olive oil to keep the noodles from sticking.

Tip

You can enjoy this dish warm or cold, depending on the season and your preference.

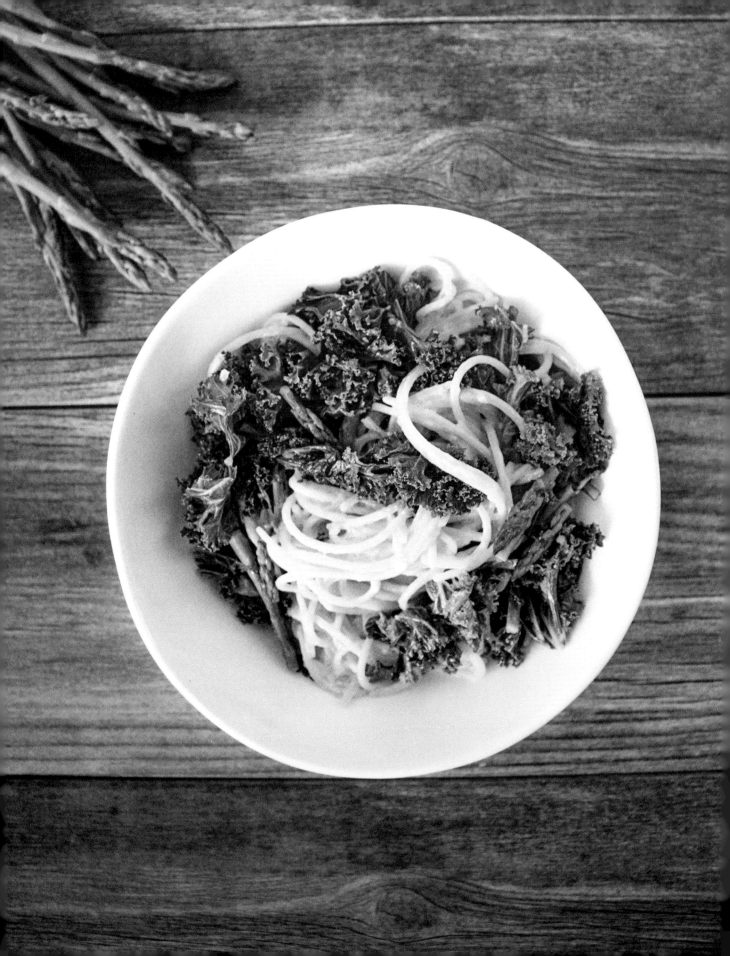

Spaghetti Alfredo

Cheesy noodles are the ultimate comfort food, and making alfredo sauce low in histamine is really easy. Mascarpone cheese takes the place of the heavy cream and Parmesan, so the finished dish is a bit lighter than the original. If you want to lighten it more, use zucchini noodles instead of gluten-free spaghetti. Pasta made of quinoa and rice will boost the protein content even more and will add even more flavor.

····· CROWD PLEASER · VEGETARIAN ·····

PREP TIME: 10 minutes • COOK TIME: 10 minutes • TOTAL TIME: 20 minutes

1 (12-ounce) package
    gluten-free spaghetti
extra-virgin olive oil
vegetables of choice
1 clove garlic
1 tablespoon butter
8 ounces mascarpone
    cheese
½ teaspoon salt

1. In a large pot over medium heat, cook the pasta according to the package instructions, drain, and set aside.

2. In a large skillet over medium heat, sauté the vegetables in a little oil for about 10 minutes, depending on size and desired doneness. Set aside.

3. Mince the garlic.

4. When the pasta has almost finished cooking, combine the butter and garlic in a large skillet over medium heat and sauté for 2–3 minutes.

5. Add the mascarpone cheese and salt to the garlic butter and mix for about 2 minutes to combine thoroughly.

6. Add the pasta to the skillet and toss to coat the noodles.

7. Serve the vegetables on top of the noodles or add them to the skillet and toss to coat.

Note

For the sautéed veggies, try asparagus, broccoli, kale, mushrooms.

Tip

If you want to make this dish into more of a macaroni and cheese, use 1 small onion instead of garlic and gluten-free macaroni or penne.

Variation

To make this low FODMAP, substitute 1 tablespoon garlic oil (or 1 tablespoon of olive oil steeped with 1 clove of garlic for 10 minutes) for the garlic.

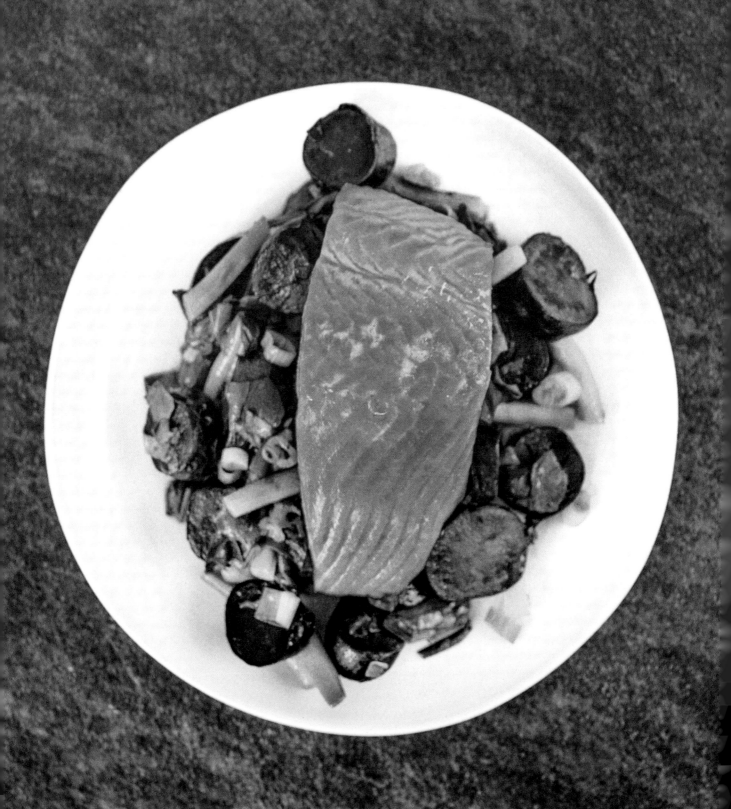

Salmon & Vegetable Medley

The salmon in this dish contains lots of omega-3s, and the purple potatoes contrast beautifully with the color of the fish. Swiss chard is rich in vitamin K, C, magnesium, and potassium. All of the antioxidants in the green and purple veggies also help protect against heart disease and inflammation.

····· HIGH PROTEIN · SUPERFOOD ·····

PREP TIME: 5 minutes · COOK TIME: 20 minutes · TOTAL TIME: 25 minutes

2 tablespoons butter, divided

2 tablespoons extra-virgin olive oil, divided

¾ teaspoon salt, divided

1 large salmon fillet (about 1 pound)

2 cups chopped green beans

2 cups chopped Swiss chard

1 cup chopped scallions

4 purple potatoes

1. In a medium sauté pan over medium heat, add 1 tablespoon butter and 1 tablespoon olive oil.

2. Rub ¼ teaspoon of salt into the salmon fillet, place the salmon, flesh side down, in the pan, and cook for 5 minutes.

3. Flip the fillet and cook for 5 more minutes on the other side. The fish has finished cooking when the flesh flakes easily.

4. Meanwhile, in another sauté pan, add the beans, Swiss chard, scallions, and ¼ teaspoon of salt with remaining 1 tablespoon butter and 1 tablespoon olive oil. Sauté for 5–10 minutes or until tender.

5. Wash the potatoes, poke holes in them, wrap each in a wet paper towel, and microwave on high for 4 minutes.

6. Slice each potato into small rounds. Add the rounds and ¼ teaspoon of salt to the pan of vegetables for the last 2 or 3 minutes of sautéing.

7. Serve the salmon over the vegetables.

Tip

Try this dish with the Basil Dressing (page 225).

Grilled Chicken & Vegetables

Grilling is one of the fastest ways for making weeknight dinners come together. If you have veggies such as asparagus that don't grill as easily, fold them into a packet of aluminum foil and steam them alongside the chicken and other grill-friendly vegetables. Using thin-cut chicken will save a lot of time because it will cook in about the same amount of time as the vegetables.

····· CROWD PLEASER · DAIRY FREE · HIGH PROTEIN ·····

PREP TIME: 5 minutes · COOK TIME: 20 minutes · TOTAL TIME: 25 minutes

1 clove garlic, minced

1 tablespoon minced rosemary

1 tablespoon minced chives

2 tablespoons extra-virgin olive oil, divided

2 pinches salt, divided

4 thin-cut chicken breasts, about 1 pound

1 bunch asparagus, tough ends removed

2 zucchini

2 red, yellow, or orange bell peppers

1. Preheat the grill to medium heat.

2. Combine garlic, rosemary, chives, 1 tablespoon of oil, and pinch of salt. Place the chicken in the herb mixture to marinate and set aside while you prepare the vegetables.

3. Remove the woody ends of the asparagus and discard them.

4. Cut the zucchini lengthwise in ⅓-inch slices and cut the bell peppers into quarters.

5. Wrap the asparagus stalks in an aluminum-foil packet and seal it.

6. Rub the zucchini and peppers with the remaining 1 tablespoon of olive oil and a pinch of salt.

7. Grill the chicken and vegetables for 5–6 minutes.

8. Carefully flip them over and cook for another 5–6 minutes or until the vegetables and chicken cook through.

> **Tip**
>
> *Try this dish with the Basil Dressing (page 225) or Mango Sauce (page 231).*

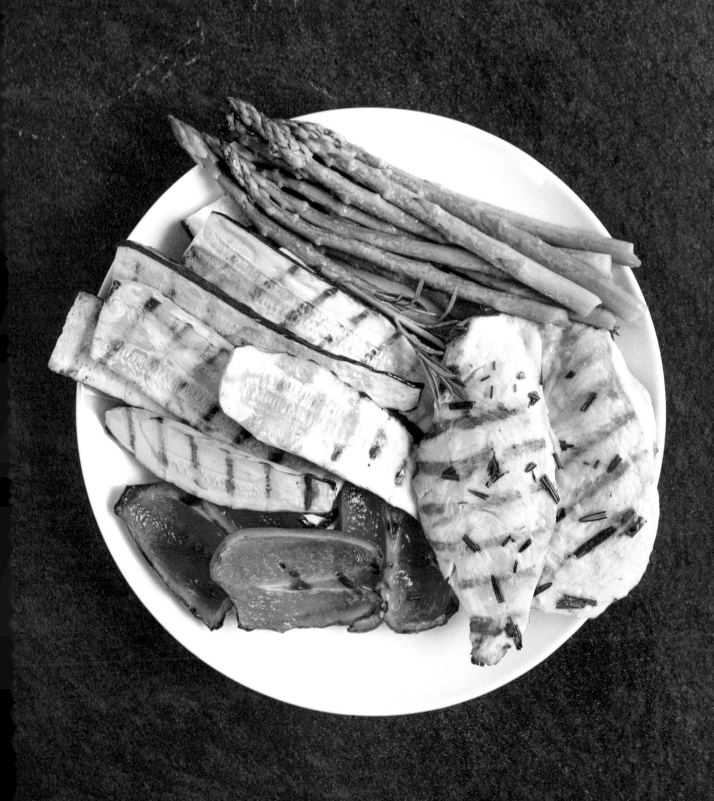

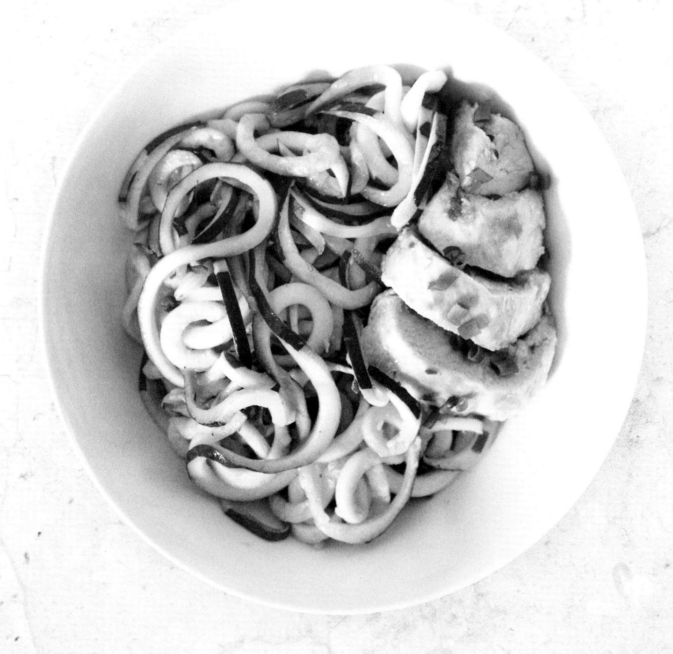

Zucchini Noodles & Chicken Scampi

Spiralizers are an amazing kitchen tool, and zucchini noodles are one of my favorites to make with the machine. They make an otherwise heavy, high-carb meal taste light. Don't boil them like regular noodles, though! If you do, they'll turn to mush. Just sauté them with a little olive oil and garlic. Thin-cut chicken breasts cook up super fast, so they're great for a quick weeknight meal.

····· DAIRY FREE · HIGH PROTEIN · KID FRIENDLY ·····

PREP TIME: 10 minutes · COOK TIME: 15 minutes · TOTAL TIME: 25 minutes

6 zucchinis

3 cloves garlic

4 tablespoons extra-virgin olive oil, divided, plus more for serving

1 pound thin-cut boneless, skinless chicken breasts

salt

¼ cup fresh chives for garnish

1. Using a vegetable spiralizer, make the zucchini noodles and set aside.

2. Mince the garlic.

3. Preheat 2 large skillets over medium heat. Add 2 tablespoons of olive oil to each skillet.

4. In the first skillet, add ⅓ of the minced garlic, chicken breasts, and salt. Sauté the chicken about 5 minutes on each side or until the chicken cooks through.

5. At the same time, in the second skillet, add the zucchini noodles and remaining ⅔ of the minced garlic. Cook the noodles about 10 minutes, until tender.

6. Serve by placing the chicken atop the zucchini noodles, then drizzle with olive oil and garnish with chives.

Tip

Spiralize a double batch of zucchini noodles so you have them on hand for another meal. They will keep in the refrigerator for 2–3 days.

Black Bean Burgers

Veggie burgers in general and black bean burgers in particular make great staples for lunch and dinner. Make a big batch and freeze them for when you're short on time. Black beans are rich in resistant starches that feed the bacteria in our microbiome, helping to keep the flora there happy and healthy, and they contain lots of antioxidants and protein.

····· CROWD PLEASER · GREAT SNACK · HIGH PROTEIN · VEGAN ·····

PREP TIME: 10 minutes • COOK TIME: 20 minutes • TOTAL TIME: 30 minutes

1 clove garlic

1 sweet onion

3 tablespoons extra-virgin olive oil, divided

2 cups black beans (cooked from scratch or defrosted from frozen)

½ cup rolled oats

1 teaspoon paprika

½ teaspoon oregano

salt and pepper

FOR SERVING

½ red onion

6 leaves Bibb leaf lettuce

Ketchup (page 229)

1. Mince the garlic and petite dice the onion.

2. In a medium pan over medium heat, sauté the garlic and onion in 2 tablespoons of olive oil until tender.

3. Transfer the garlic and onion to a bowl and add the black beans, oats, paprika, oregano, and salt and pepper to taste.

4. Using a potato masher, mash the bean mixture until it combines well.

5. Form the bean mixture into six patties

6. In a preheated skillet over medium heat, sauté the patties in 1 tablespoon of olive oil for 3–4 minutes.

7. Flip and cook for another 3–4 minutes.

8. While the burgers finish cooking, slice the red onion into ¼-inch rings for serving.

9. Serve the burgers in a lettuce wrap with the onion and Ketchup.

> **Variation**
>
> *For a heartier version, have the burgers on an Oatmeal Roll (page 46) with Caramelized Onions (page 227).*

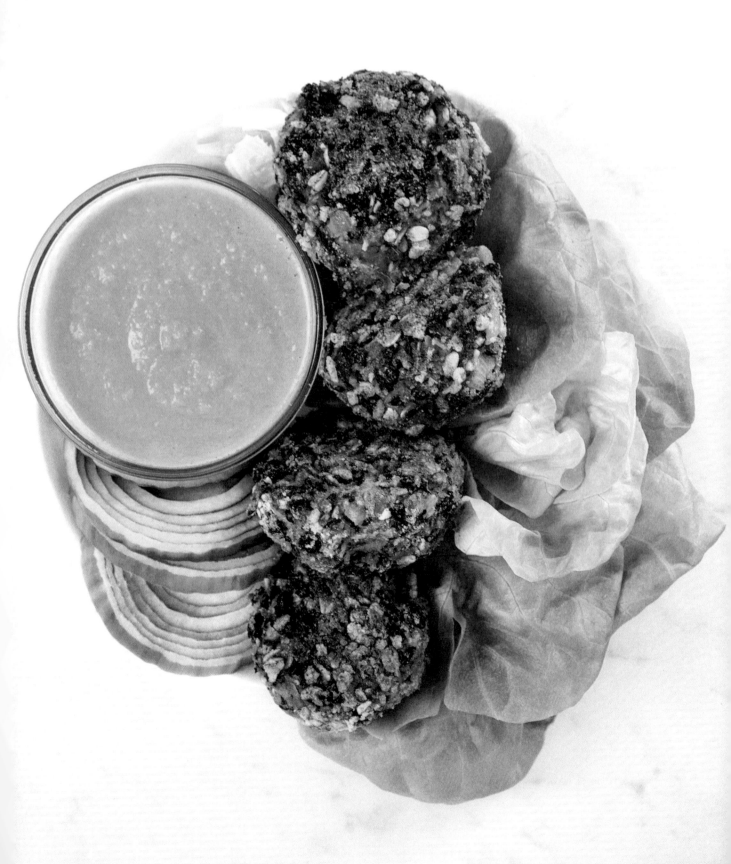

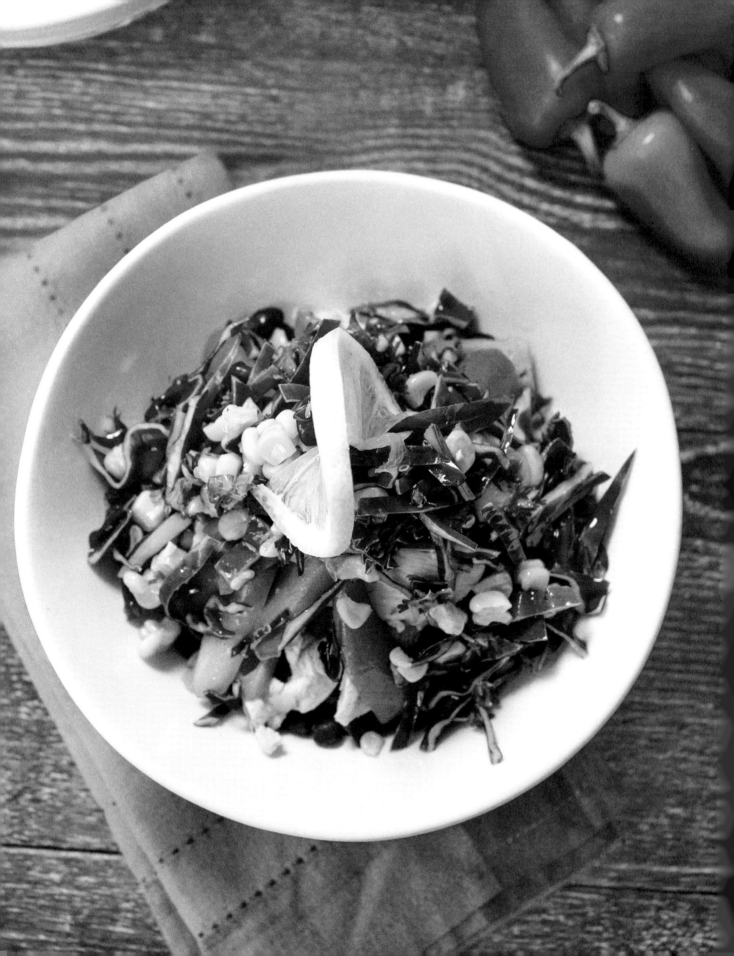

Fajita Chicken Rice Bowl

Mexican food always works well as a quick meal for busy weeknights. The trick is to make large batches of beans, rice, and quinoa ahead of time and freeze them in single portions to make meal prep go even faster. Just microwave the single portions for 2–3 minutes on high until they thaw, and you're ready to go! This dish tastes delicious when made half with basmati rice and half with quinoa. The combination gives it a nice light flavor but also boosts the protein content.

····· CROWD PLEASER · DAIRY FREE · HIGH PROTEIN · SUPERFOOD ·····

PREP TIME: 10 minutes · COOK TIME: 20 minutes · TOTAL TIME: 30 minutes

4 cups water

1 cup dry basmati rice

1 cup dry quinoa

1 clove garlic

1 red, yellow, or orange bell pepper

12 ounces boneless, skinless chicken breast

1 sweet onion

1 tablespoon extra-virgin olive oil

juice of ½ lemon

1 teaspoon dried oregano

½ teaspoon cumin

1 pinch salt

1 cup cooked black beans

CABBAGE SLAW

1 cup organic corn (defrosted from frozen)

2 cups chopped purple cabbage

2 tablespoons chopped fresh parsley

1 tablespoon extra-virgin olive oil

1 teaspoon lemon juice

1 pinch salt

1. First make the rice and quinoa. In a medium pot filled with water, add the rice and quinoa. Bring to a boil, reduce heat to low, and simmer for 20 minutes. Alternately, if you batched the ingredients ahead of time, defrost 2 servings of rice and 2 of quinoa in the microwave.

2. Mince the garlic and slice the bell pepper, chicken breast, and onion.

3. Preheat a large skillet over medium heat, then add the olive oil.

4. Add the peppers, chicken, onions, lemon juice, oregano, garlic, cumin, and salt to the skillet. Cook for 15 minutes until the onions and peppers become tender and the chicken cooks through. Add a little water if necessary during cooking to prevent excessive browning and to keep the chicken moist.

5. Meanwhile, make the slaw. In a small bowl, add the corn, cabbage, parsley, olive oil, lemon juice, and salt. Mix thoroughly to combine.

6. In a large serving bowl, layer the rice mixture on the bottom, then the black beans and the chicken-and-pepper mixture, and top with the cabbage slaw.

MAKES 4 SERVINGS

Mushroom Rosemary Chicken

This savory chicken dish is packed with histamine-lowering ingredients. Mushrooms help regulate the immune system and add a wonderful depth of flavor to many dishes. Rosemary reduces histamine release from mast cells, and it also smells and tastes amazing.

····· CROWD PLEASER · HIGH PROTEIN ·····

PREP TIME: 10 minutes • COOK TIME: 20 minutes • TOTAL TIME: 30 minutes

12 ounces white cremini mushrooms
1 clove garlic
1 sweet onion
2 tablespoons extra-virgin olive oil
1 pound thin-cut boneless, skinless chicken breasts
2 tablespoons tapioca starch
½ cup water
2 tablespoons finely chopped fresh rosemary
½ teaspoon salt
1 tablespoon butter
Cauliflower Mash (page 133)

1. Slice the mushrooms, mince the garlic, and dice the onion.
2. In a medium skillet over medium heat, add the mushrooms, garlic, onion, and olive oil and sauté for 3–4 minutes.
3. Meanwhile, dredge the chicken breasts in the tapioca starch and add to the pan.
4. Add the water, rosemary, and salt, cover, and poach the chicken in the mushroom sauce for about 8 minutes.
5. Flip the chicken and stir the sauce. Cook, uncovered, for another 6–8 minutes or until the chicken cooks through.
6. With 2 minutes of cooking remaining, add the butter and stir the sauce again.
7. Serve with the Cauliflower Mash.

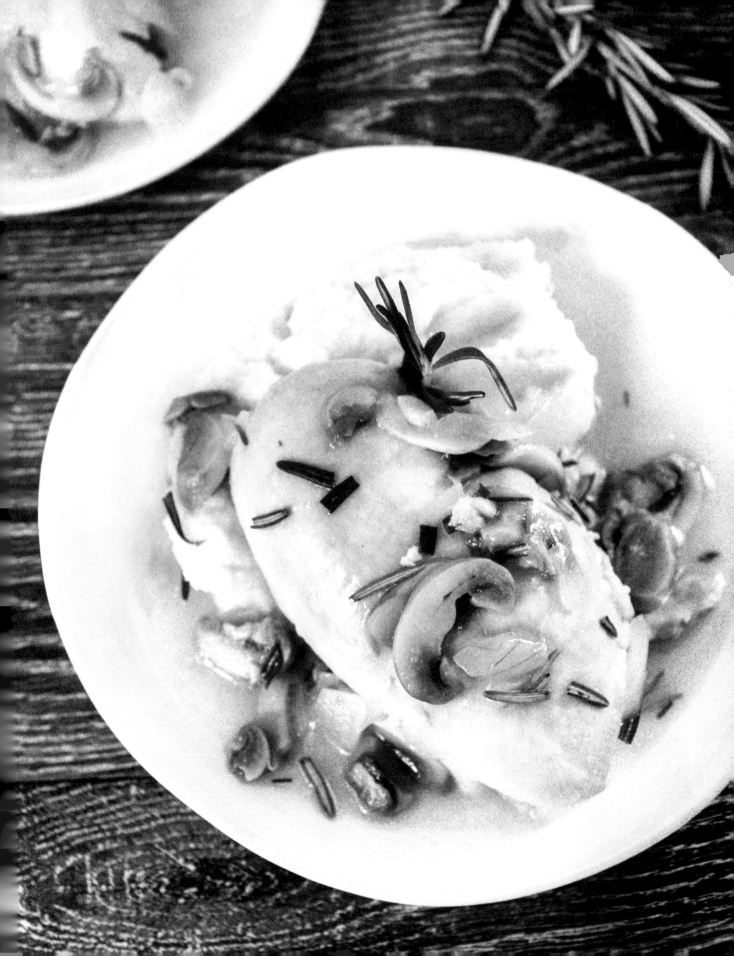

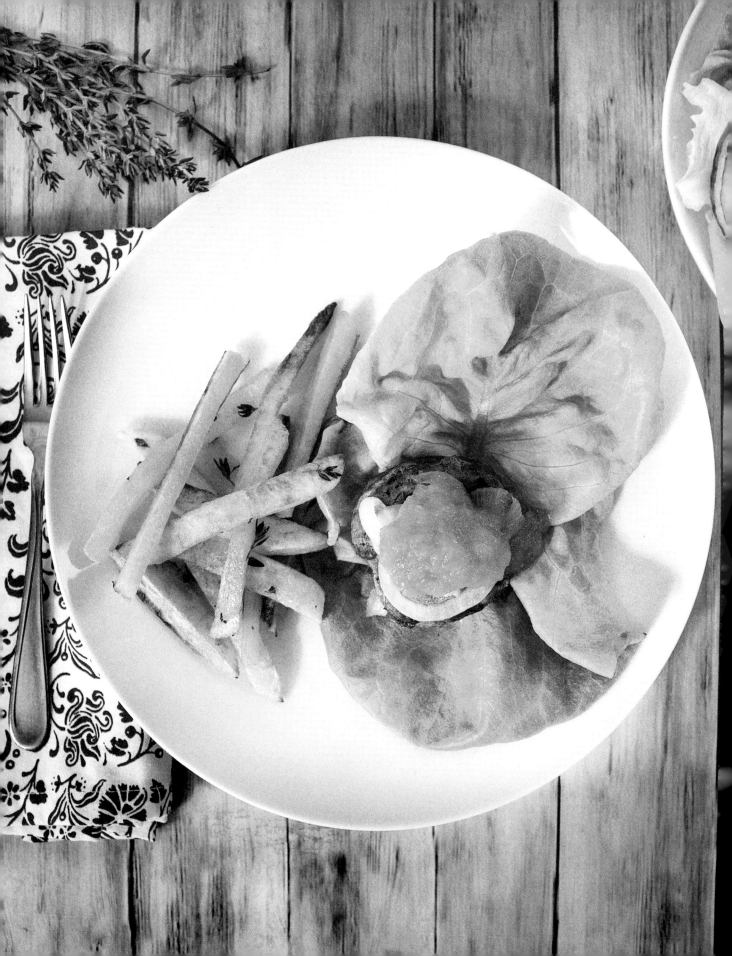

Lettuce-Wrapped Burgers

Yes, you can have burgers on an anti-inflammatory diet. The key is not to have them too often and to make them in a way that limits the amount of histamine they contain. Remember, the goal isn't to deny ourselves but to make tasty food that feeds the body and soul. Everybody loves burgers, and this recipe keeps them heart-healthy by using turkey or chicken. Wrapping the burger in lettuce decreases the amount of carbs and adds more nutrition. The onions and ketchup contain a ton of quercetin and add a nice zing to the burger.

····· CROWD PLEASER · DAIRY FREE · HIGH PROTEIN · KID FRIENDLY ·····

PREP TIME: 10 minutes • COOK TIME: 20 minutes • TOTAL TIME: 30 minutes

2 tablespoons extra-virgin
   olive oil, divided
salt and pepper
1 pound freshly ground
   turkey or chicken
1 sweet onion
4 large butter or Bibb
   lettuce leaves
Ketchup (page 229)
Thyme Garlic Fries
   (page 145)

1. Preheat a grill to medium heat.

2. Add 1 tablespoon olive oil and salt and pepper to taste to the burger meat. Form into patties.

3. Grill the burgers for about 8–10 minutes on each side, until they cook through.

4. Meanwhile, slice the onion.

5. In a skillet over medium heat, add 1 tablespoon olive oil and the sliced onion and sauté for about 10 minutes, stirring occasionally.

6. Top with the onions and Ketchup, wrap in lettuce, and serve with Thyme Garlic Fries.

> ### Variation
>
> *Substitute the Ketchup for Cranberry Chutney (page 228), and you have an easy, fresh, new take on Thanksgiving.*
>
> *Turkey or chicken is the healthier option, but you can make this with grass-fed ground beef as well.*

Vegetable Coconut Curry

This veggie-rich coconut curry has lots of anti-inflammatory ingredients, including turmeric, ginger, onions, peppers, and broccoli. Again, you can freeze this recipe in batches to thaw for quick meals. The vegetables provide lots of vitamin C and phytochemicals.

····· SUPERFOOD · VEGAN ·····

PREP TIME: 10 minutes • COOK TIME: 20 minutes • TOTAL TIME: 30 minutes

1 cup dry basmati rice

1 cup dry quinoa

4 cups water

1 head broccoli

1 zucchini

1 red bell pepper

1 cup fresh snap peas

2 scallions

1 sweet onion

1 tablespoon grated ginger

½ teaspoon turmeric

1 (13½-ounce) can
   coconut milk

salt

1. First make the rice and quinoa. In a medium pot, add 4 cups of water. Add the rice and quinoa. Bring to a boil, reduce heat to low, and simmer for 20 minutes. Alternately, if you batched the ingredients ahead of time, defrost 2 servings of rice and 2 of quinoa in the microwave.

2. Cut the broccoli into florets and slice the zucchini and bell pepper into ¼-inch pieces.

3. Destem and destring the snap peas and chop the scallions.

4. Slice the onion (last to avoid kitchen tears).

5. In a skillet over medium heat, add all of the vegetables and simmer with the ginger, turmeric, coconut milk, and salt to taste for about 15 minutes or until the sauce thickens and all of the vegetables become tender.

6. Serve over quinoa and rice.

> Note
>
> *Drink a cup of holy basil tea, which goes great with curry dishes, for some extra anti-inflammatory power.*
>
> Tip
>
> *Freeze any extra rice-quinoa mixture or vegetable curry in resealable freezer bags for up to 3 months.*

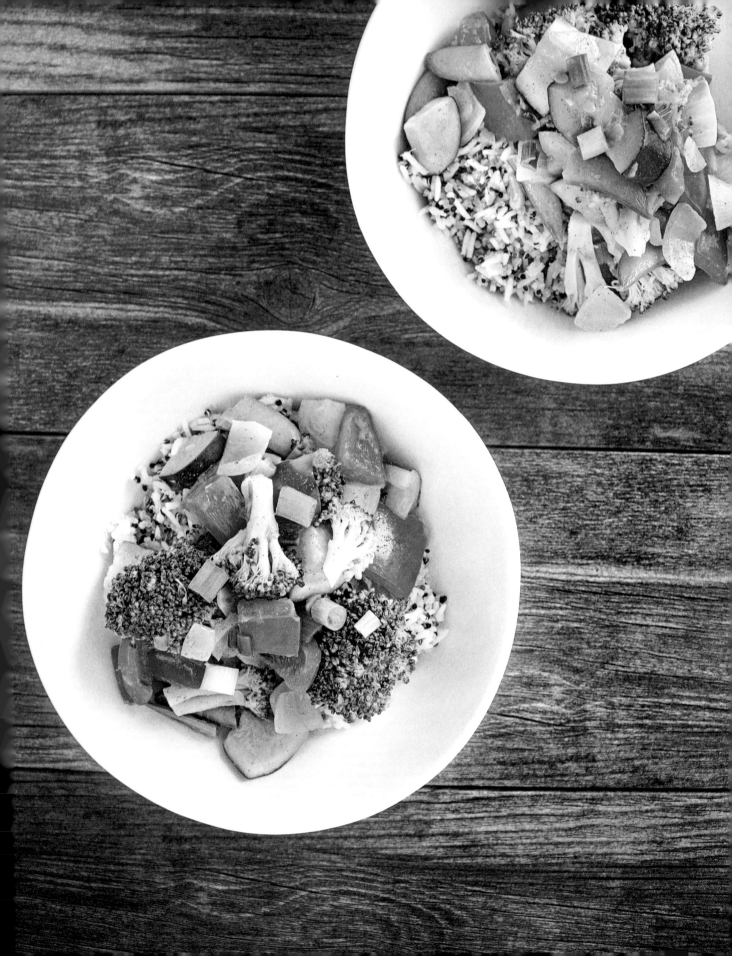

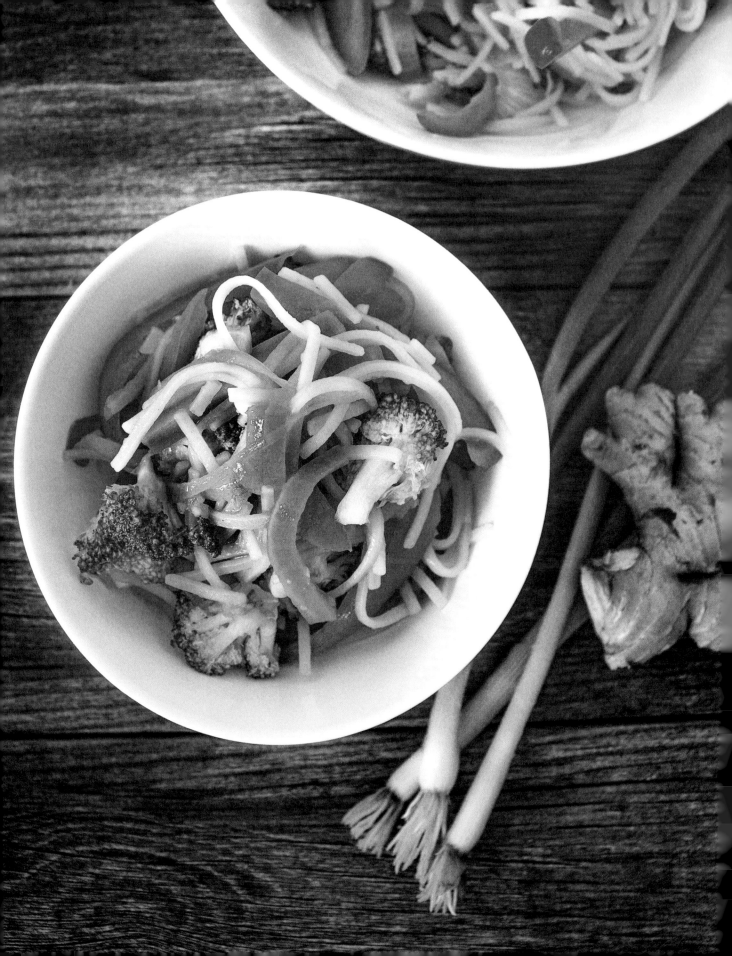

Asian Stir-Fry Noodles

Soy sauce has lots of histamine, so it's a no-go for an anti-inflammatory, low-histamine diet. This light noodle dish still packs lots of great taste, though. The ginger, garlic, and onion add histamine-stabilizing flavonoids, and bell peppers are a great source of vitamin C, which supports DAO production.

····· SUPERFOOD · VEGAN ·····

PREP TIME: 15 minutes • COOK TIME: 15 minutes • TOTAL TIME: 30 minutes

1 large head broccoli

3 large carrots

1 red bell pepper

1 sweet onion or 1 bunch
  scallions

2 tablespoons grated ginger

2 cloves garlic, minced

1 tablespoon sesame oil or
  extra-light olive oil

1 (12-ounce) package
  straight-cut rice noodles

2 tablespoons brown sugar
  or coconut sugar

½ teaspoon salt

1. Chop the broccoli into florets, peel and julienne the carrots, slice the bell pepper into strips, and mince the garlic.

2. Thinly slice the onion (last to avoid kitchen tears).

3. In a large pan over medium heat, combine the vegetables, ginger, and garlic and sauté in the sesame oil for 10 minutes or until the vegetables become tender.

4. Meanwhile, heat a large pot of water to boiling, add the noodles, and cook for 8–10 minutes.

5. Drain the noodles and rinse them with hot water.

6. Add the sugar and salt to the vegetables and cook for 1–2 minutes, stirring until they dissolve.

7. Add noodles to the vegetables and stir to combine.

> **Tip**
>
> *For more protein, serve this dish with sautéed salmon.*

Mockaroni & Cheese

This creamy pasta dish looks and tastes just like macaroni and cheese—but without the cheese. The white beans add more creaminess and more protein to this dish, and this is a great way to hide some beans in your or your kiddos' diet. They can't tell what's in there, and kids of all ages love mac and cheese. The sweet potatoes and carrots provide a boost of vitamin A and carotenoid compounds, and quinoa-based gluten-free noodles will increase the protein power here as well.

····· CROWD PLEASER · KID FRIENDLY · VEGETARIAN ·····
PREP TIME: 15 minutes • COOK TIME: 15 minutes • TOTAL TIME: 30 minutes

2 carrots

1 sweet potato

1 sweet onion

2 tablespoons extra-virgin
olive oil

1½ cups water

½ cup white beans, cooked
fresh or defrosted from
frozen

2 tablespoons butter

½ teaspoon salt

1 (14-ounce) package gluten-
free macaroni

1. Peel and dice the carrots, sweet potato, and onion.

2. In a medium saucepan, add the carrots, sweet potato, onion, olive oil, and water. Simmer for 15 minutes or until the vegetables become tender.

3. Add the white beans, butter, and salt. Use an immersion blender to blend into a thick and creamy sauce.

4. Meanwhile, in another pot, cook the noodles according to the package directions. Reserve a few tablespoons of the cooking water before draining the noodles.

5. In a large bowl, combine the sweet potato sauce, noodles, and the reserved pasta water. Toss to coat evenly.

> **Note**
>
> *You can use navy, cannellini, or great northern beans for this recipe.*

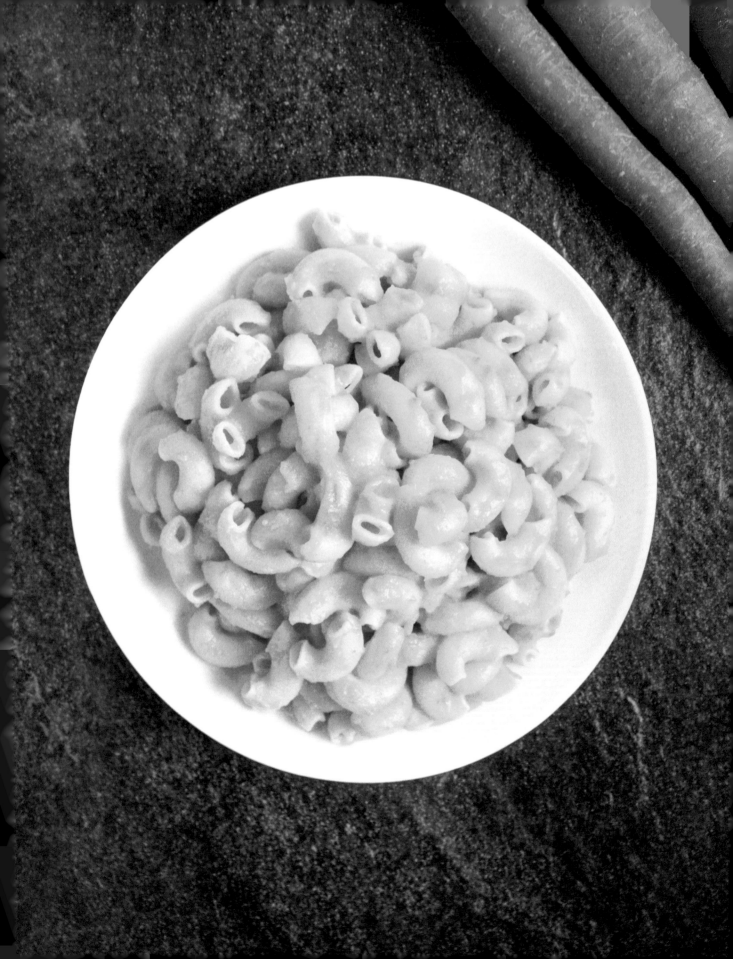

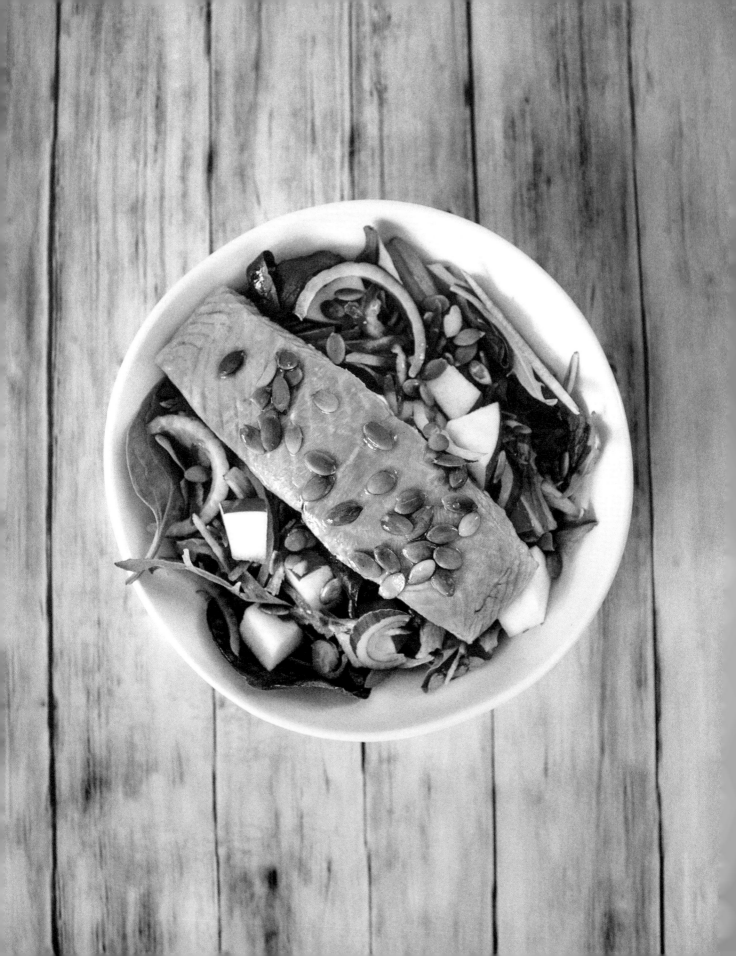

Salmon Apple Salad

Fish can have high levels of histamine if not handled properly. Try to get fish frozen at sea whenever possible and buy it frozen (not thawed). You also want to cook it from frozen at home rather than thawing it first. If you live in a seaside community, the catch at your local fish market is likely fresh and well handled. The omega-3 fatty acids in salmon help reduce inflammation in the body, and on top of that, this salad boasts tons of natural quercetin, zinc, vitamins A and C, and folate.

····· DAIRY FREE · HIGH PROTEIN ·····

PREP TIME: 15 minutes • COOK TIME: 15 minutes • TOTAL TIME: 30 minutes

1 red apple

lemon juice

2 carrots

1 pound fresh salmon

1 tablespoon extra-virgin olive oil

8 cups mesclun

¼ cup raw pumpkin seeds

½ red onion, sliced

DRESSING

1 tablespoon lemon juice

1 tablespoon maple syrup

3 tablespoons extra-virgin olive oil

1 pinch salt

1. Preheat the oven to 400°F.

2. Core and dice the apple and toss it with a little lemon juice.

3. Shred the carrots with a vegetable peeler.

4. On a baking sheet prepared with 1 teaspoon olive oil, roast the salmon for 15 minutes until the flesh flakes with a fork. Divide into four servings.

5. Meanwhile, prepare the salad in a large bowl by tossing the greens with the shredded carrots, diced apples, pumpkin seeds, and red onion.

6. To make the dressing, thoroughly combine the lemon juice, maple syrup, remaining olive oil, and salt.

7. Fill a large plate or bowl with the salad, top with 1 serving of the salmon, and drizzle with the dressing.

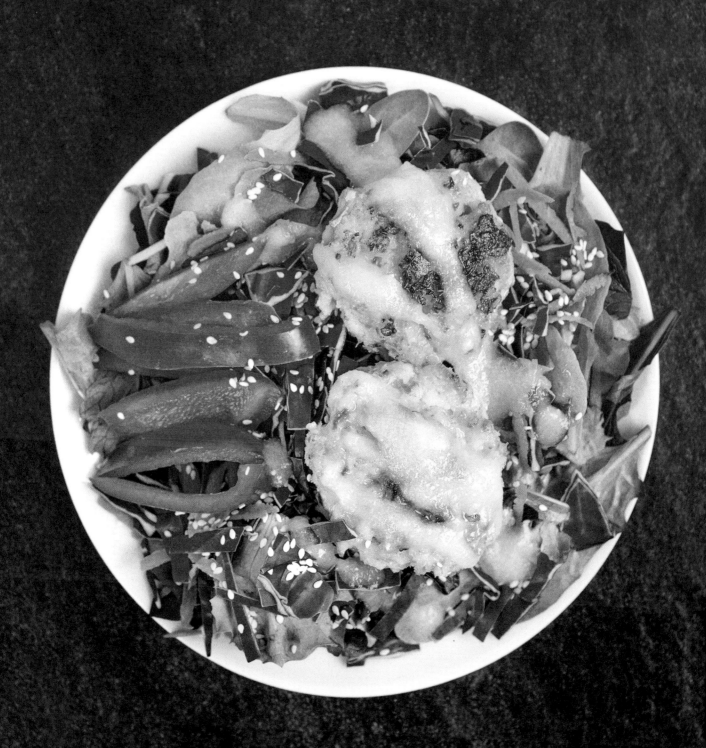

Cod Cakes with Mango Sauce

You can make these tasty, tropical fish cakes with cod or haddock, and they come together quickly with a food processor. The mangos, peppers, and scallions brighten up the white fish and add lots of vitamins to this recipe. Serve with the Super Salad with Sesame Garlic Dressing (page 86). The light, nutty sesame dressing will add some nice depth to the bright mango sauce and the fish.

····· DAIRY FREE · HIGH PROTEIN · SUPERFOOD ·····

PREP TIME: 15 minutes · COOK TIME: 20 minutes · TOTAL TIME: 35 minutes

¼ cup fresh mango cubes

⅛ cup sliced red bell pepper

2 scallions

1 pound cod or other whitefish

1 egg

1 pinch salt

¾ cup crushed crispy rice cereal, divided

2 tablespoons extra-light olive oil

Mango Sauce (page 231)

1. Preheat the oven to 400°F.

2. Prepare the mango cubes and red pepper and chop the scallions.

3. In the bowl of a food processor, add the mango cubes, bell pepper, and scallions. Pulse until they break into small pieces.

4. Add the cod and pulse until the fish breaks up but doesn't form a paste.

5. In a medium bowl, thoroughly combine the fish mixture, egg, salt, and ¼ cup crushed crispy rice cereal.

6. Form the fish batter into 6 small cakes and dredge each in the remaining ½ cup crushed cereal.

7. In a skillet over medium heat, add the olive oil and cook the cakes for about 3–4 minutes on each side, until golden.

8. Place the cakes on a baking sheet and bake them for 10 minutes or until the middles completely cook through.

9. While the cakes are baking, make the Mango Sauce.

10. Serve the cakes on a bed of greens with your favorite veggies.

Tip

Crush the crispy rice cereal in a resealable plastic bag either by hand, with a meat tenderizer, or with a rolling pin until it forms fine crumbs.

Basil & Garlic Salmon with Sautéed Greens

This simple salmon recipe is teeming with flavor from the garlic and basil. Swiss chard is rich in betalains, a phytonutrient commonly found in beets that acts as a strong anti-inflammatory agent and boosts detoxification in the body. Swiss chard is also rich in vitamins K, A, and C.

····· DAIRY FREE · HIGH PROTEIN · SUPERFOOD ·····

PREP TIME: 15 minutes • COOK TIME: 20 minutes • TOTAL TIME: 35 minutes

6 large leaves basil

1 clove garlic

1 teaspoon extra-virgin olive oil

4 (4-ounce) salmon fillets

1 pinch salt

GREENS

1 clove garlic

2 large bunches Swiss chard

1 tablespoon olive oil

1 pinch salt

1. Preheat the oven to 375°F.

2. Chop the basil and mince the garlic.

3. Drizzle a baking sheet with the olive oil and place the salmon fillets in the center.

4. Top the fillets with the basil, garlic, and salt.

5. Bake for about 20 minutes, until the salmon flesh flakes easily with a fork.

6. Meanwhile, prepare the greens. Mince the garlic and sauté the Swiss chard and garlic in the olive oil and a pinch of salt for 8 minutes or until tender.

7. Serve the salmon over the greens.

> **Variation**
>
> *To make this recipe low FODMAP, substitute the garlic for a drizzle of garlic-infused or garlic-steeped oil.*

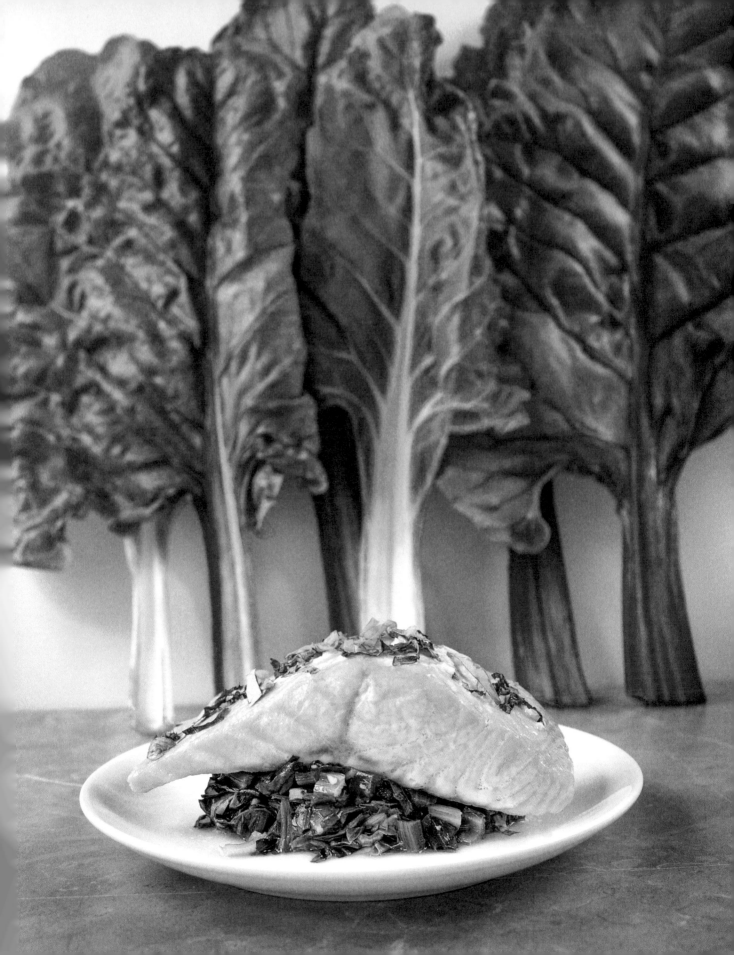

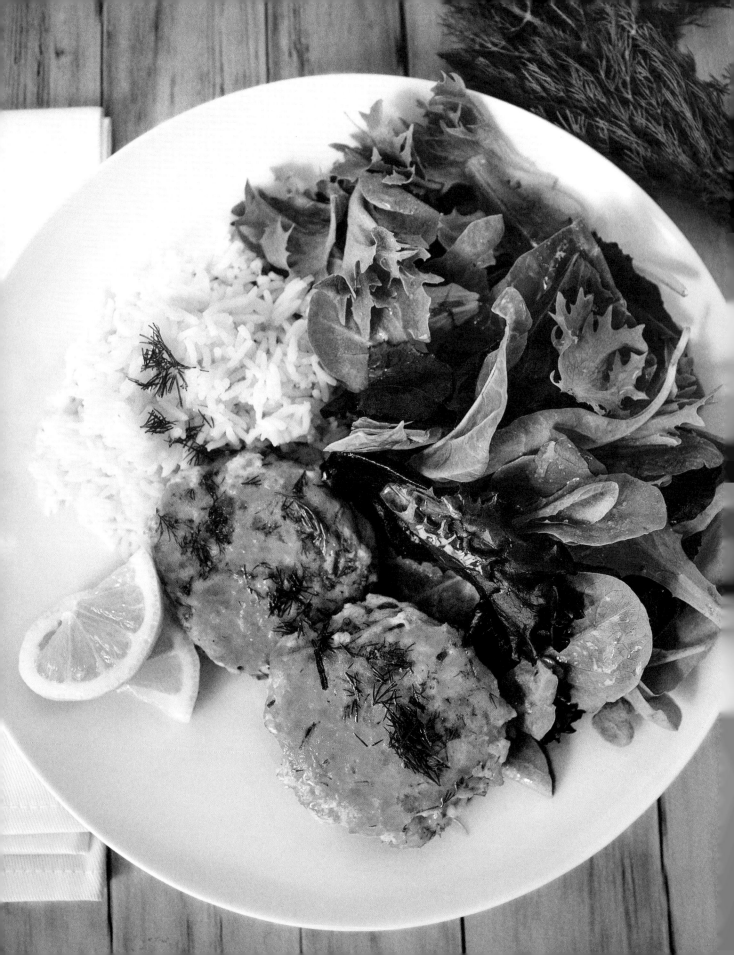

Salmon Cakes with Dill Butter

If handled well, fish can be friendly to a low-histamine diet. Look for frozen-at-sea options or purchase fresh from your local fish market for the best quality and lowest histamine. Omega-3s are very important for reducing inflammation, and one of best ways to season salmon is with dill, lemon juice, and chives. The herbs brighten the salmon and change the texture of what otherwise would taste like plain old fish.

····· GREAT SNACK · HIGH PROTEIN · SUPERFOOD ·····

PREP TIME: 15 minutes • COOK TIME: 20 minutes • TOTAL TIME: 35 minutes

2 cups dry basmati rice

1 pound fresh salmon, skin removed

1 egg

3 tablespoons chopped dill

2 tablespoons chopped chives

juice of ½–1 lemon

¼ cup crushed crispy rice cereal

1 pinch salt

3 tablespoons extra-virgin olive oil

8 cups salad greens

DILL BUTTER

2 tablespoons butter, room temperature

2 tablespoons chopped fresh dill

1 pinch salt

> **Tip**
>
> *Crush the cereal in a resealable plastic bag by hand or with a rolling pin.*

1. Cook the basmati rice according to the package directions.

2. Preheat the oven to 400°F.

3. In a food processor, pulse the salmon until the flesh just breaks into small pieces. You don't want it to form a paste.

4. Add the egg, herbs, lemon juice, crushed cereal, and salt to the food processor and pulse 1–2 more times to combine the ingredients.

5. Preheat a skillet to medium heat and add the olive oil.

6. Form the salmon mixture into 4 cakes and cook them in the skillet for 4 minutes on each side, until golden brown.

7. Transfer the patties to a baking sheet and bake the cakes for 10 minutes to cook them all the way through.

8. While the rice is cooking and the cakes are baking, make the dill butter. Combine the butter, dill, and salt in a small bowl and mix with a fork. Slather it on the salmon cakes just before serving.

9. Serve the cakes with mixed greens and rice.

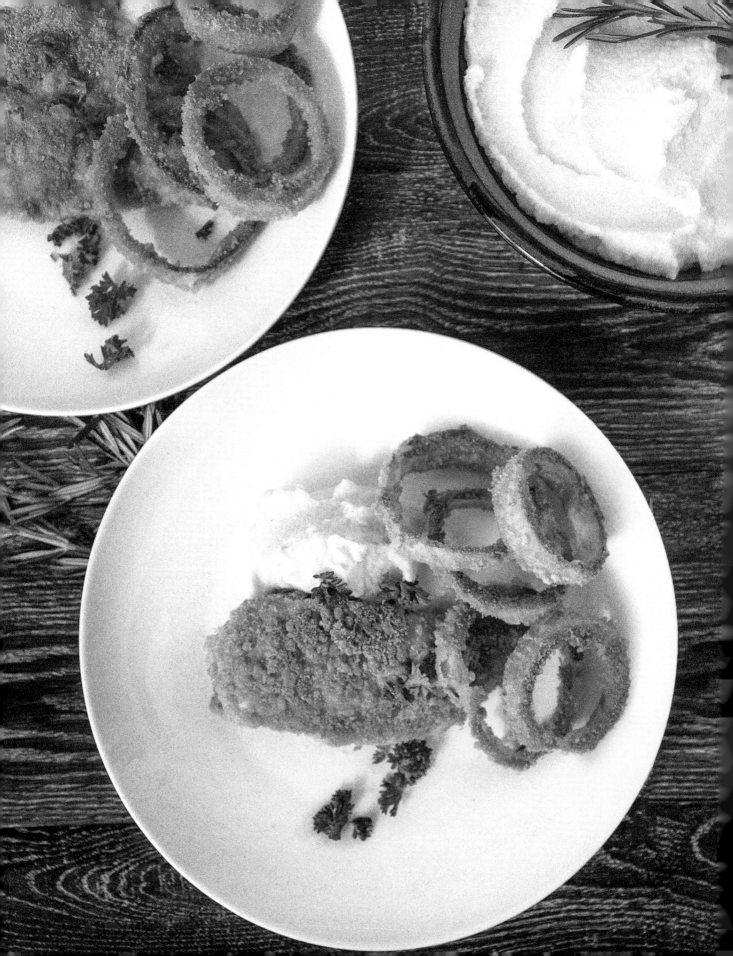

Oven-Fried Chicken

Sometimes you just crave fried food. This recipe gives you a nice, crispy crust on the chicken without drowning it in frying oils like restaurants do. The key to achieving that crunch is sautéing the chicken in olive oil, then baking it in the oven.

····· CROWD PLEASER · DAIRY FREE · HIGH PROTEIN · KID FRIENDLY ·····

PREP TIME: 20 minutes • COOK TIME: 15 minutes • TOTAL TIME: 35 minutes

¼ cup All-Purpose Flour Blend (page 28)

½ teaspoon salt

¼ teaspoon paprika

4 thin-cut boneless, skinless chicken breasts

1 egg

1 cup crushed crispy rice cereal

4 tablespoons extra-light olive oil, divided

Onion Rings (page 142)

Cauliflower Mash (page 133)

1. Preheat the oven to 400°F.

2. On a shallow plate, mix together the All-Purpose Flour Blend, salt, and paprika.

3. Dredge the chicken breasts in the flour mixture and set aside.

4. Beat the egg and pour it onto another shallow plate.

5. Add the crushed cereal to a third shallow plate.

6. In a large skillet over medium heat, add 2 tablespoons olive oil.

7. While the oil is heating, dip each flour-dredged chicken breast first in the egg, then in the cereal. Coat on all sides and place on a clean plate.

8. Cook the chicken in the skillet for 3–4 minutes on each side until each side becomes crispy and golden.

9. Place the chicken pieces on a baking sheet and bake for 5–6 minutes.

10. Serve with Onions Rings and Cauliflower Mash for a truly indulgent, healthier version of a comfort meal.

> **Variation**
>
> *Try a corn-based cereal for a different flavor.*

Zucchini Latkes with Applesauce

Latkes are delicious, but they're also heavy. The zucchini in this recipe lightens the calorie load and the carbs and adds more nutrition. Parsley, a strong anti-inflammatory agent, also adds a nice, fresh taste to this dish. You can't have sour cream on a low-histamine diet, but apples contain quercetin, so applesauce is no problem.

····· DAIRY FREE · GREAT SNACK · KID FRIENDLY · VEGETARIAN ·····
PREP TIME: 10 minutes • COOK TIME: 30 minutes • TOTAL TIME: 40 minutes

4 yellow potatoes

1 sweet onion

1 zucchini

2 tablespoons chopped fresh parsley

½ cup All-Purpose Flour Blend (page 28)

½ teaspoon salt

1 egg

4 tablespoons extra-light olive oil, divided

Applesauce (page 224)

1. Preheat the oven to 375°F.

2. Peel the potatoes and the onion.

3. Use a food processor to shred the potatoes, onion, and zucchini quickly. Squeeze the extra water from the shredded vegetables by hand.

4. In a large bowl, combine the potatoes, onion, zucchini, parsley, All-Purpose Flour Blend, salt and egg.

5. Preheat a large skillet over medium heat. Add 2 tablespoons of olive oil.

6. Add ¼-cup scoops of the latke mixture to the skillet and cook for about 5 minutes. Cook 4 latkes at a time.

7. Flip the latkes, pressing them gently with a spatula for even frying, and cook for another 5 minutes.

8. Place the first batch of latkes on a baking sheet in the oven to continue crisping while you cook the second batch.

9. Add the remaining 2 tablespoons olive oil to the pan and cook the remaining latkes as above.

10. While the latkes are cooking, make the Applesauce.

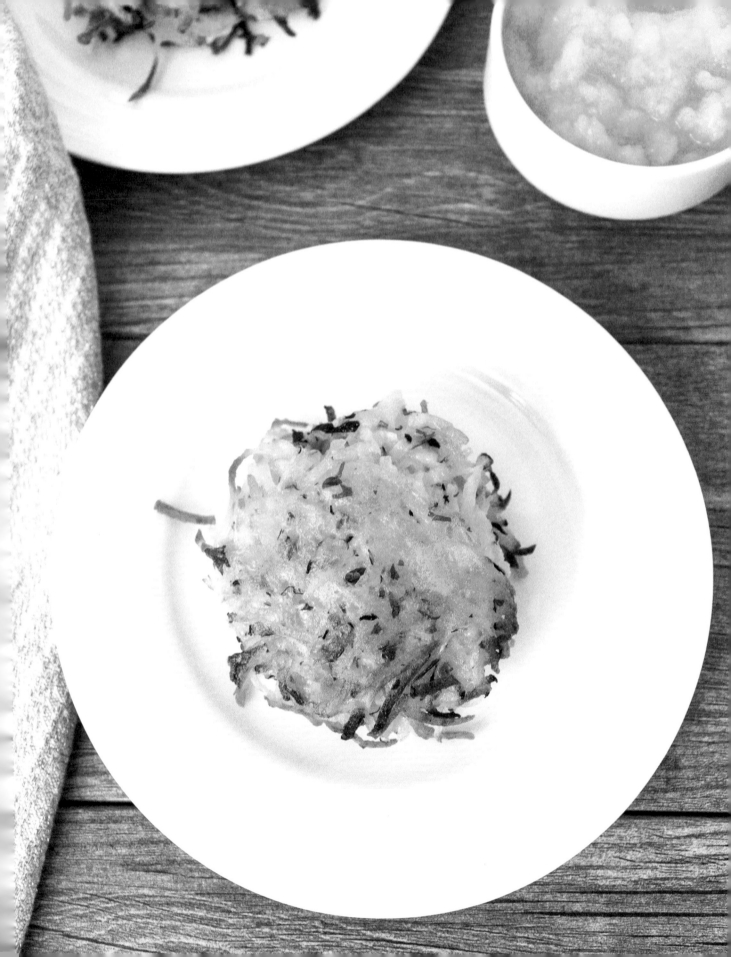

Mushroom Risotto

MAKES 6 SERVINGS

This recipe tastes just as rich and creamy as a true Italian risotto, but it contains no wine, store-bought broth, or aged cheese, so it has a much lower histamine content. The mushrooms help stimulate the immune system and add a wonderful flavor, making this good-for-you comfort food.

····· CROWD PLEASER · KID FRIENDLY · VEGETARIAN ·····

PREP TIME: 10 minutes • COOK TIME: 30 minutes • TOTAL TIME: 40 minutes

12 ounces white cremini mushrooms

2 cloves garlic

1 sweet onion

6 cups Vegetable Broth (page 237)

3 tablespoons extra-virgin olive oil, divided

2 cups dry Aborio rice

8 ounces mascarpone cheese

2 tablespoons butter

salt

1. Slice the mushrooms, mince the garlic, and dice the onion.

2. In a medium pot, heat the broth until boiling.

3. Meanwhile, in a large saucepan over medium heat, add 2 tablespoons of the olive oil, the onions, and garlic and sauté for about 3 minutes.

4. Add the rice and 1 cup of the hot broth to the saucepan. Stir as the broth is absorbed, for about 5 minutes.

5. Meanwhile, in a skillet, sauté the mushrooms in the remaining 1 tablespoon of olive oil until they cook through, about 8 minutes. Set aside.

6. Continue stirring the rice mixture over medium-low heat as the broth is absorbed into the rice.

7. Add more broth when the previous broth is absorbed. This will take about 20 minutes.

8. Once the rice has cooked (slightly al dente), add the mascarpone cheese, mushrooms, butter, and salt to taste and stir thoroughly to combine.

> **Tip**
>
> *This dish pairs well with the Rosemary Sea Salt Brussels Sprouts (page 136).*

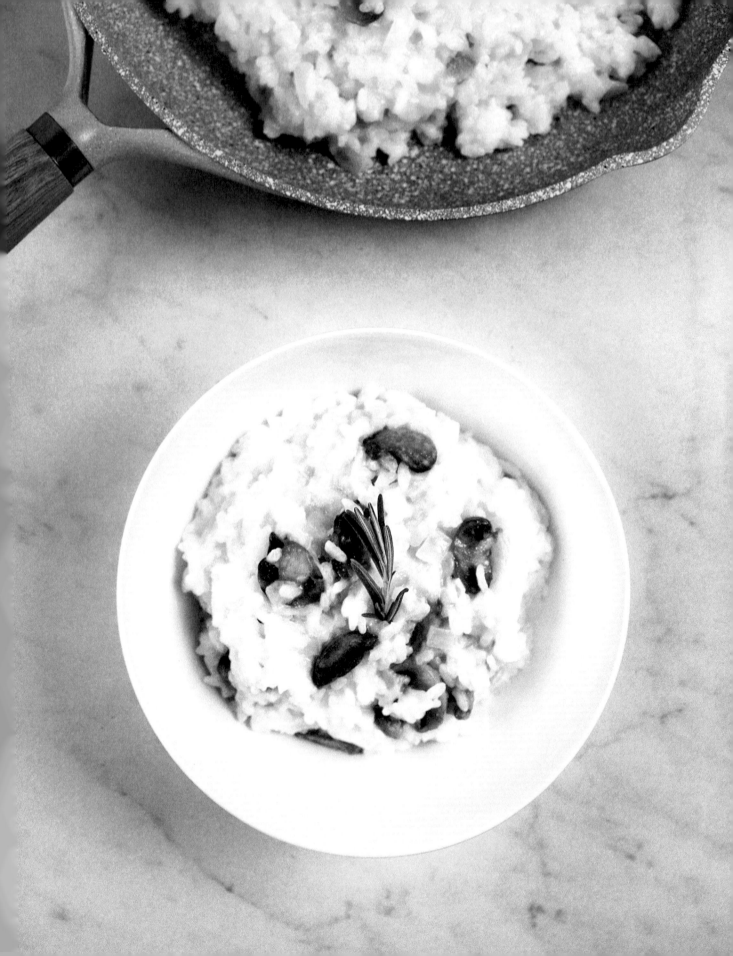

Ginger Vegetable Fried Rice with Sautéed Bok Choy

Fried rice doesn't sound healthy, but it can be if you make it the right way at home and avoid the high-histamine soy sauce. Bok choy, also known as Chinese cabbage, is rich in glucosinolates, which are sulfur-containing compounds found to reduce the risk of cancer. Bok choy is also rich in vitamins K, C, and A.

····· CROWD PLEASER · GREAT SNACK · VEGETARIAN ·····

PREP TIME: 10 minutes • COOK TIME: 30 minutes • TOTAL TIME: 40 minutes

4 cups cooked brown or
  white rice
½ cup chopped green beans
1 tablespoon grated ginger
½ cup diced carrots
1 sweet onion
4 tablespoons sesame oil,
  divided
1 cup frozen peas
½ teaspoon salt, plus more
  to taste
2 cups baby bok choy (whole,
  bottom stem removed for
  presentation)
4 eggs

1. Prepare the rice, green beans, ginger, and carrots and dice the onion.

2. In a large skillet over medium heat, add 2 tablespoons sesame oil and sauté the green beans, ginger, carrots, and onion for about 8 minutes or until tender.

3. Add the rice, frozen peas, and salt and sauté for 2–3 minutes, then set aside.

4. Meanwhile, in a skillet over medium heat, add 1 tablespoon sesame oil, the bok choy, and salt to taste. Sauté for about 5 minutes or until the bok choy turns golden and soft.

5. In another skillet over medium heat, add 1 tablespoon of sesame oil and the eggs.

6. Scramble the eggs until they cook through and break into little chunks, add them to rice-and-vegetable mixture, and stir to combine thoroughly.

7. Serve the fried rice alongside the sautéed bok choy.

> ### Variation
>
> *For a richer, vegetarian version of this dish, use half butter and half sesame oil.*

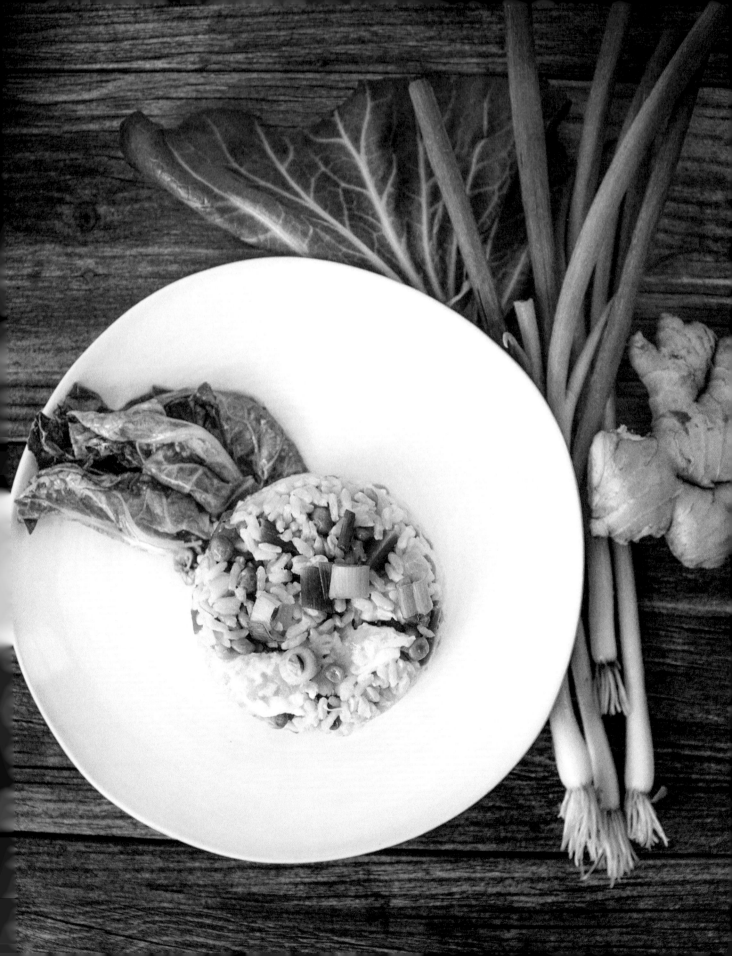

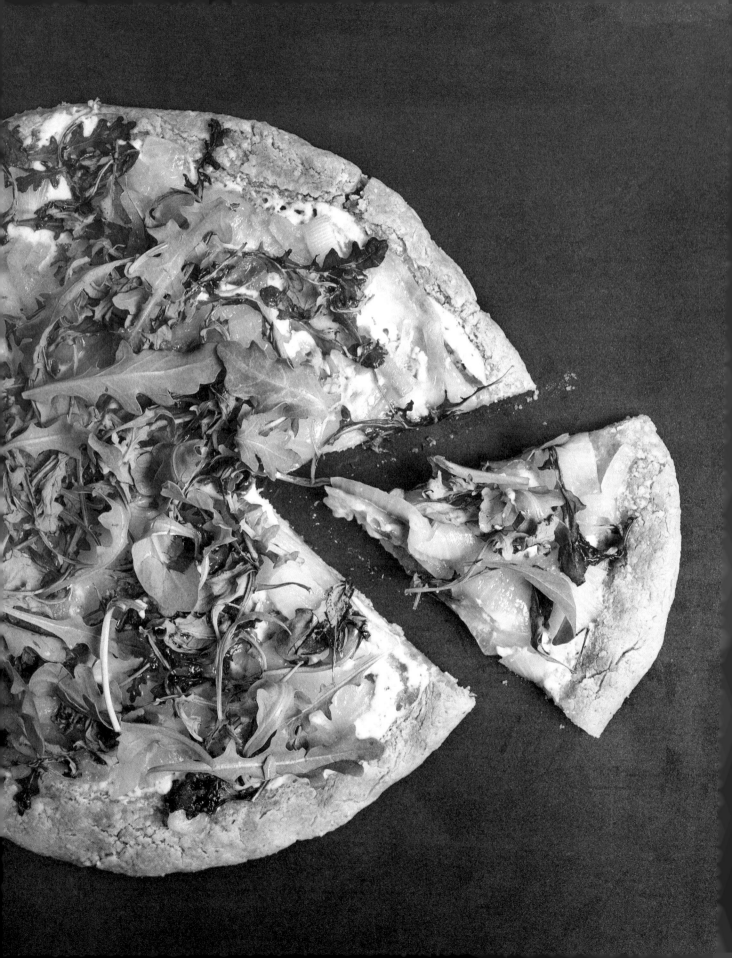

Caramelized Onion & Arugula Pizza

This yummy, flavorful flatbread is great for dinner or as an appetizer for a larger group. It's also a great way to keep eating your favorite foods on an anti-inflammatory diet. The creamy mascarpone cheese acts as a low-histamine white sauce, and the onions, a powerful anti-inflammatory rich in quercetin, boost the flavor. Homemade oat flour amps the depth, fiber, and nutrition of the recipe.

····· CROWD PLEASER · KID FRIENDLY · VEGETARIAN ·····

PREP TIME: 20 minutes • COOK TIME: 20 minutes • TOTAL TIME: 40 minutes

DOUGH:

2 tablespoons extra-virgin olive oil, plus 1 tablespoon for greasing
⅔ cup rolled oats
2 cups All-Purpose Flour Blend (page 28)
½ teaspoon salt
1 teaspoon baking powder
3/4 cup water

TOPPINGS

8 ounces mascarpone cheese
½ cup Caramelized Onions (page 227)
1 cup arugula

1. Preheat the oven to 400°F.

2. Prepare a baking sheet with 1 tablespoon of olive oil.

3. In a food processor, pulse the rolled oats into ½ cup of oat flour.

4. In a medium bowl, combine the flours, salt, 2 tablespoons of olive oil, baking powder, and water into a dough and knead into a ball 5–6 times.

5. Let the dough rest, covered on the counter for 5 minutes.

6. Spread the dough by hand on the baking sheet to about ½-inch thickness.

7. Top the dough with the mascarpone, then the Caramelized Onions.

8. Bake for 10 minutes, add the arugula on top, and cook for another 10 minutes or until the crust turns golden brown.

Spaghetti Squash Pasta with Chicken Meatballs & Pomodoro Sauce

Spaghetti squash makes a great substitute for pasta, gluten-free or otherwise, if you're trying to reduce your carb intake, and it's super easy to make chicken or turkey meatballs at home in your food processor. My family couldn't tell the difference between the ones below and our old store-bought standby turkey-burger meatballs. The pomodoro sauce has a higher onion-to-tomato ratio than traditional tomato sauce, providing more quercetin and histamine-fighting compounds.

····· DAIRY FREE · HIGH PROTEIN · KID FRIENDLY ·····

PREP TIME: 15 minutes • COOK TIME: 30 minutes • TOTAL TIME: 45 minutes

2 tablespoons extra-virgin olive oil, plus more for greasing and serving

1 sweet onion

2 tablespoons chopped fresh basil, plus more for garnish

1 teaspoon dried oregano

1 large leaf Swiss chard, stems removed

1 pound fresh chicken breasts, cut into 1-inch pieces

1 egg

½ cup crushed crispy rice cereal or crushed rice crackers

salt

1 (5 lb.) spaghetti squash (yields 6 cups of "noodles")

Pomodoro Sauce (page 233)

1. Preheat the oven to 375°F and prepare a baking sheet with 1 tablespoon olive oil.

2. Quarter the onion, and in the bowl of a food processor, pulse the onion, basil, oregano, and Swiss chard until minced.

3. In a skillet over medium heat, add 1 tablespoon olive oil and sauté the Swiss chard mixture for 3–4 minutes or until tender.

4. In the food processor, with the blade already spinning, add the chicken breasts, pulsing until the meat breaks into small pieces but doesn't form a paste.

5. In a large bowl, combine the meat and the basil mixture, then add the egg, cereal or cracker crumbs, and salt to taste.

6. Form the meat mixture into 12 (1-inch) balls and bake on the prepared pan for 20–25 minutes.

7. Meanwhile cut the squash in half and remove the seeds.

8. Place the squash halves, flesh side up, in a glass baking dish with ½ inch of water and cover. Microwave for 15 minutes on high until the squash is fork tender.

9. String the squash flesh out into noodles, add the meatballs to them, and top with Pomodoro Sauce.

10. Garnish with fresh basil and a drizzle of olive oil.

Variation

You can make this recipe with 1 pound gluten-free spaghetti instead. Prepare it according to the package instructions while the meatballs are baking. If you can't tolerate tomatoes, try the No-mato Pomodoro Sauce (page 232) instead.

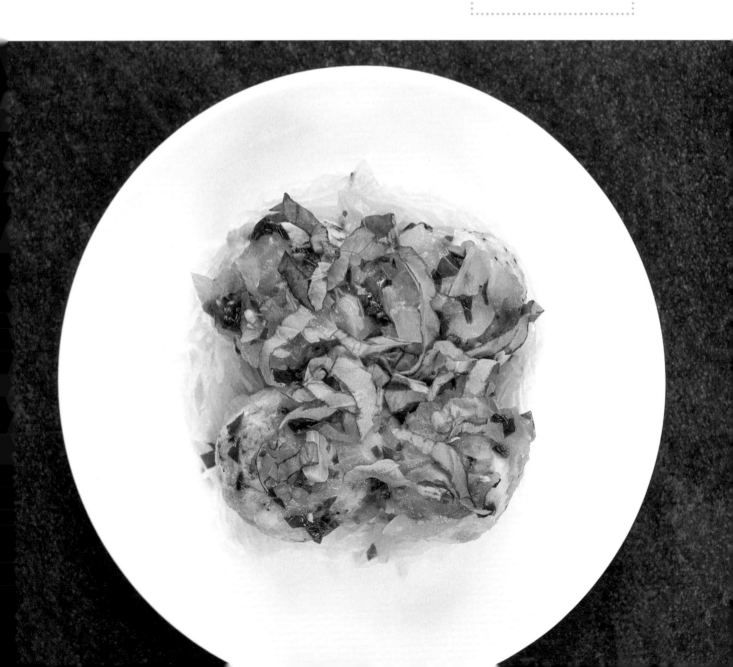

Sesame Chicken

Looking for a healthy version of General Tso? Cutting the soy sauce can make it hard to create a flavorful dish, but try making this at home. The vegetables are all anti-inflammatory, and their juices mixed with the brown sugar make a sweet-and-savory sauce. Black rice adds a nice nutty flavor and has histamine-lowering properties to boot.

····· CROWD PLEASER · DAIRY FREE · HIGH PROTEIN · SUPERFOOD ·····

PREP TIME: 20 minutes · COOK TIME: 35 minutes · TOTAL TIME: 55 minutes

2 cups dry black rice

4¼ cups water, divided

2 cloves garlic

1-inch piece ginger

1 head broccoli

2 tablespoons extra-light olive oil

1 pound boneless, skinless chicken breasts

4 tablespoons tapioca starch, divided

2 tablespoons sesame oil

1 red bell pepper

1 sweet onion

2 tablespoons brown sugar or coconut sugar

½ teaspoon salt

1. In a medium pot over high heat, combine the rice and 4 cups water and heat to boiling, then reduce to low heat. Cover and simmer for about 35 minutes, until the rice becomes tender. Set aside.

2. Meanwhile, mince the garlic and grate the ginger. Then cut the broccoli into florets, the chicken into ½-inch pieces, and the bell pepper and onion into thin slices.

3. In a large pot with a steamer basket, add 1 inch of water and the broccoli and cook, covered, for about 10 minutes, until tender. Set aside.

4. In a medium skillet over medium heat, add 2 tablespoons of olive oil.

5. Coat the chicken chunks with 2 tablespoons of the tapioca starch, then pan-fry them for 2–3 minutes on each side, until the chicken turns golden and cooks through.

6. In a small skillet over medium heat, add the sesame oil, garlic, pepper, and onion and stir-fry for 2–3 minutes.

7. Add the ginger, brown sugar, and salt to the small skillet. Simmer the vegetables for 3–4 minutes or until tender.

8. In a bowl, combine the remaining 2 tablespoons of tapioca starch with the remaining water and mix.

9. Add the tapioca slurry to the vegetable sauce and simmer for 1 more minute so the sauce thickens.

10. Add the chicken to the sauce and stir thoroughly to coat.

11. Serve the chicken with 1 cup of the rice and ¼ of the broccoli per portion.

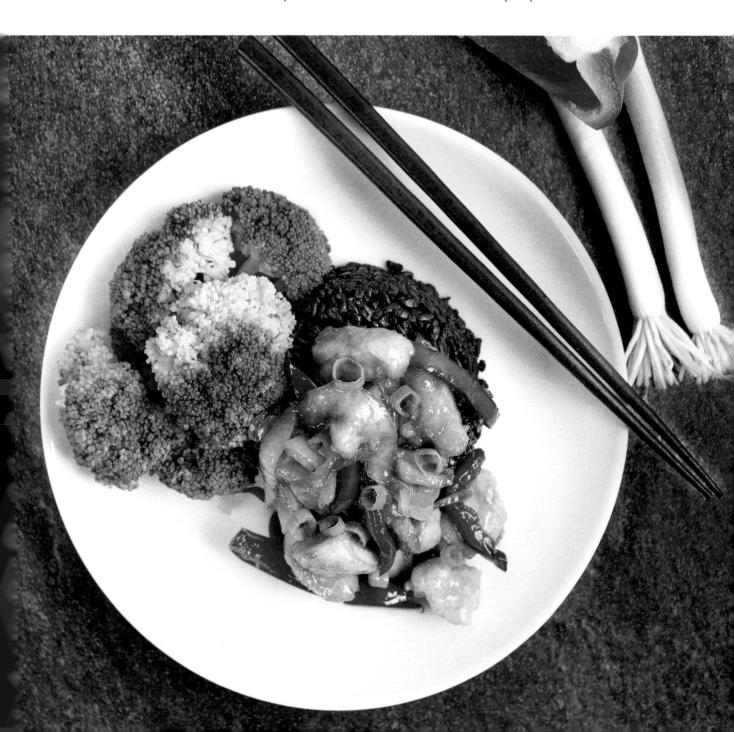

Beef Tenderloin with Herb Butter

Conventional red meat has high levels of omega-6 fatty acids because the cows eat a diet primarily consisting of corn. But a cow's natural diet is grass, and the meat from grass-fed cows has more naturally occurring omega-3 fatty acids in it. You can eat red meat occasionally on an anti-inflammatory diet—1–2 times per month, maximum—and for the best option buy grass-fed organic beef.

····· HIGH PROTEIN ·····

PREP TIME: 10 minutes • COOK TIME: 50 minutes • TOTAL TIME: 1 hour

8 red potatoes

1 clove garlic

3 tablespoons extra-light olive oil, divided

1 tablespoon chopped fresh rosemary, plus 2 sprigs

1 tablespoon chopped fresh thyme, plus 4 sprigs

2 pinches salt

4 (4-ounce) grass-fed, organic beef tenderloins (such as filet mignon)

2 tablespoons butter

Rosemary Sea Salt Brussels Sprouts (page 136)

1. Preheat the oven to 400°F.

2. Chop the potatoes into ½-inch chunks, and mince the garlic.

3. Toss the potatoes with 1 tablespoon each of olive oil, rosemary, thyme as well as the garlic and a pinch of salt.

4. On a baking sheet, bake the potatoes in a single later for 20–30 minutes, until they become crispy.

5. Liberally season the tenderloins with salt.

6. In a large skillet over medium heat, add 1 tablespoon olive oil. Add the tenderloins and the sprigs of rosemary and thyme.

7. Cook 5–10 minutes on each side, depending on how you like your steak cooked.

8. Baste the tenderloin with the juices in the pan every 3–4 minutes.

9. In the last 1–2 minutes of cooking, add ½ tablespoon of butter to each steak, continuing to baste with the sauce.

10. Serve with the Rosemary Sea Salt Brussels Sprouts and potatoes.

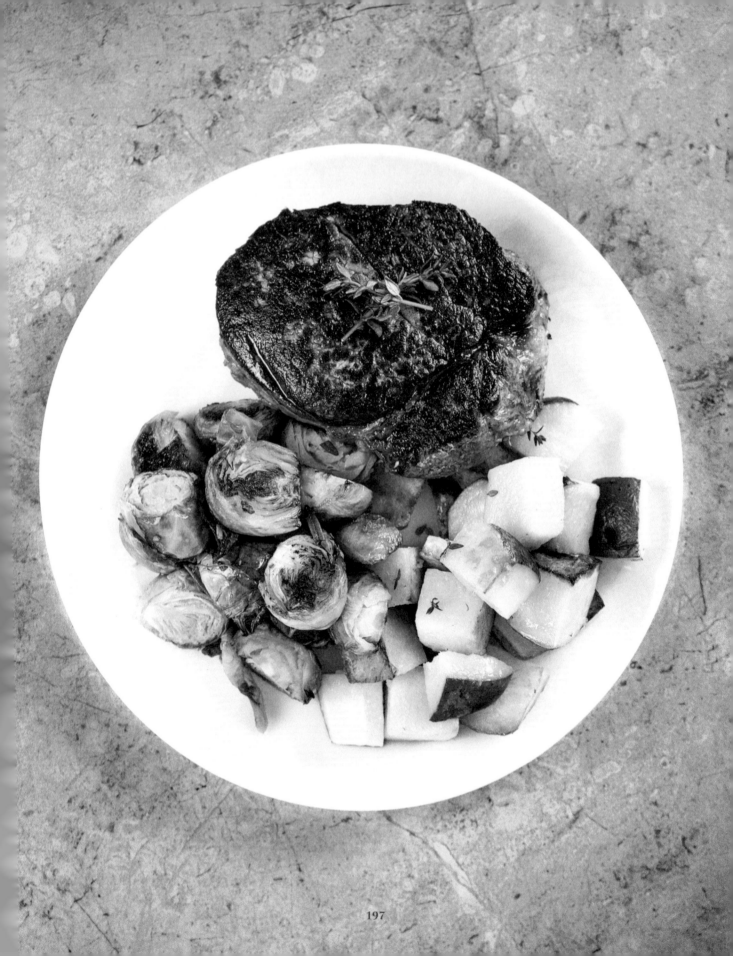

Buddha Bowl with Sunflower Dressing

Buddha bowls have become increasingly popular, and this one offers a bevy of complex carbohydrates and rich greens and herbs that serve as a balanced meal rich in anti-inflammatory ingredients. The bowl starts with a whole grain such as rice or quinoa, includes a protein such as beans, and features cooked vegetables and a seed-based dressing.

····· HIGH PROTEIN · SUPERFOOD · VEGAN ·····

PREP TIME: **20** minutes • COOK TIME: **40** minutes • TOTAL TIME: **1** hour

2 cups brown rice

4 cups water

1 large bunch kale

1 clove garlic

1 red onion

1 tablespoon extra-virgin olive oil

2 cups cooked garbanzo beans or lentils (cooked fresh or thawed from frozen)

SUNFLOWER DRESSING

juice of 1 lemon

¼ cup sunflower seeds

¼ cup fresh herbs of choice (oregano, parsley, thyme, etc.)

½ teaspoon salt

1 clove garlic

¼ cup extra-virgin olive oil

1. Add the rice and water to a large pot, cover, and bring to a boil.

2. Reduce heat to low and let simmer for 40 minutes or until all of the water is absorbed and the rice becomes tender.

3. Chop the kale, mince the garlic, and slice the onion.

4. In a medium skillet over medium heat, sauté the kale, garlic, and onions with the olive oil until tender.

5. Meanwhile, make the dressing. In the bowl of a food processor, add the lemon juice, sunflower seeds, fresh herbs, salt, garlic, and olive oil. Blend until smooth.

6. Serve the sautéed veggies over the rice and beans.

7. Divide the dressing evenly over each rice bowl.

Variation

Use different herbs, pumpkin seeds, or sesame seeds to modify the taste of the dressing.

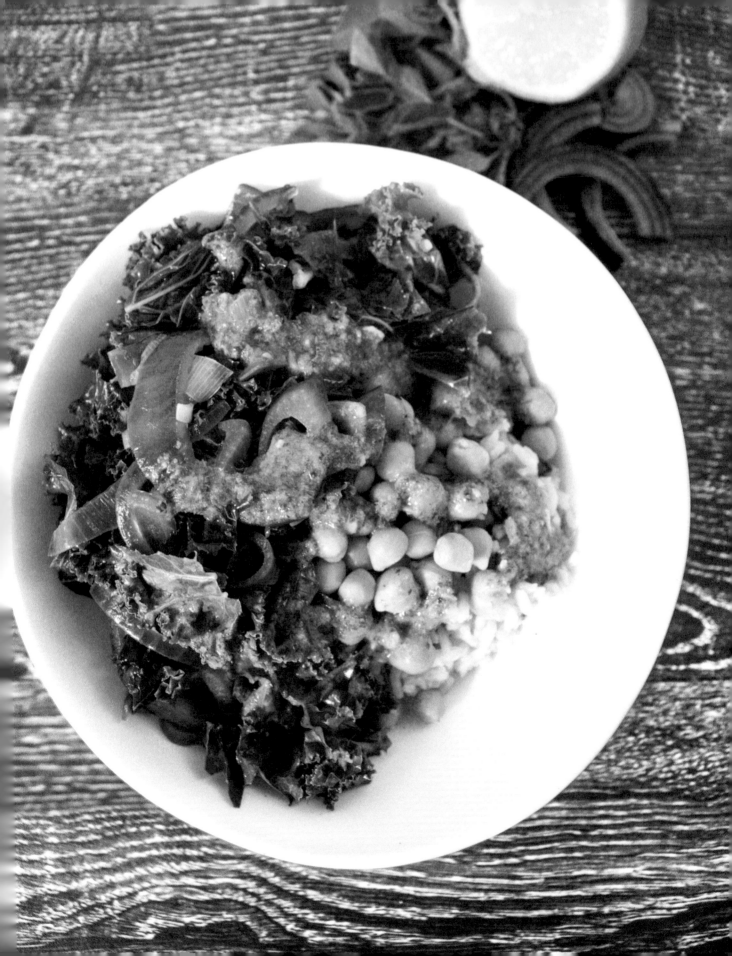

Rosemary & Garlic Chicken Breasts with Vegetables

This easy roasting dish contains loads of rosemary and garlic, which have great anti-inflammatory and histamine-lowering properties. It takes about an hour to prepare, so it's great for a Sunday meal, but the work is minimal after chopping the veggies. You can relax while it cooks. Cooking the chicken on the bone retains more moisture and flavor.

····· DAIRY FREE · HIGH PROTEIN · SUPERFOOD ·····

PREP TIME: 10 minutes • COOK TIME: 1 hour 5 minutes • TOTAL TIME: 1 hour 15 minutes

1 pound yellow, purple, and
   pink potatoes
1 sweet potato
4 carrots
2 delicata squashes
1 clove garlic
1 sweet onion
3 tablespoons extra-virgin
   olive oil, divided
salt
2 split chicken breasts
2 tablespoons chopped
   fresh rosemary

1. Preheat the oven to 400°F.

2. Chop the potatoes into 1-inch cubes; peel and chop the carrots into 1-inch cubes; deseed the delicata squashes and cut them into ⅓-inch slices; mince the garlic; and dice the onion.

3. Toss the vegetables with 2 tablespoons olive oil and a pinch of salt.

4. Place the veggies in a single layer on a baking sheet and roast them for 20 minutes.

5. Meanwhile, carefully separate the skin from the chicken breasts.

6. Rub the chicken breasts with the minced garlic, rosemary, and salt to taste.

7. When the vegetables have finished roasting, remove the baking sheet from the oven, stir them with a spatula, and lay the chicken on top of the vegetables.

8. Return the baking sheet to the oven and roast for another 45 minutes or until the chicken's internal temperature reaches 165°F as measured on a digital meat thermometer. Depending on the size of the chicken breasts, this could take up to 1 hour.

9. Plate and top the chicken with any pan drippings.

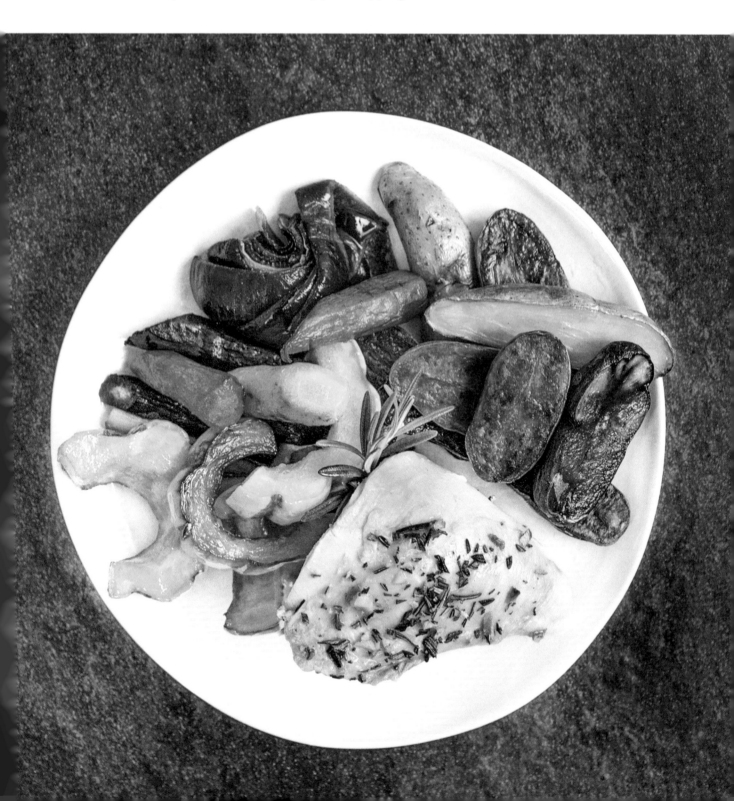

Vegetable Tart

This tart is a real treat. It works well with any vegetables, but my favorite combination is bell peppers, kale or Swiss chard, zucchini, and scallions—a midsummer harvest on a plate. For the best flavor in the crust, this recipe really needs butter, so don't substitute olive oil.

····· CROWD PLEASER · GREAT SNACK · LOW FODMAP · VEGETARIAN ·····
PREP TIME: 1 hour 10 minutes • COOK TIME: 40 minutes • TOTAL TIME: 1 hour 50 minutes

DOUGH

1 cup rolled oats
1¾ cups All-Purpose Flour Blend (page 28)
½ teaspoon salt
1 cup cold unsalted butter
⅔ cup ice water

VEGETABLES

1 yellow or orange bell pepper, chopped
1 cup chopped Swiss chard or kale, stems and central veins removed
2 cups diced zucchini
1 cup diced summer squash
1 cup diced scallions
1 tablespoon extra-virgin olive oil
½ teaspoon salt

1. First make the dough.

2. In a large bowl, combine the dry ingredients.

3. In a food processor, pulse the rolled oats into ¾ cups of oat flour.

4. Cut the butter into ½-inch cubes, then use a pastry blender to cut the butter cubes into the dry ingredients until they form pea-size lumps.

5. Slowly add the ice water and mix until the ingredients just combine into a dough.

6. Form the dough into a ball. Cover it with plastic wrap and refrigerate for at least 30 minutes and as long as overnight.

7. Preheat the oven to 375°F.

8. On a sheet of parchment paper dusted with All-Purpose Flour Blend, roll out the dough to a thickness of about ⅓ inch.

9. Place the dough and parchment paper onto a baking sheet and set aside.

10. In a medium skillet over medium heat, sauté the vegetables in the olive oil for about 10 minutes or until they completely cook through and don't have much moisture left.

11. Pour the vegetables into the middle of the tart crust, leaving a 3-inch border all around.

12. Fold the 3-inch border over the vegetables and seal the edges and any small holes.

13. Bake for about 30 minutes or until golden.

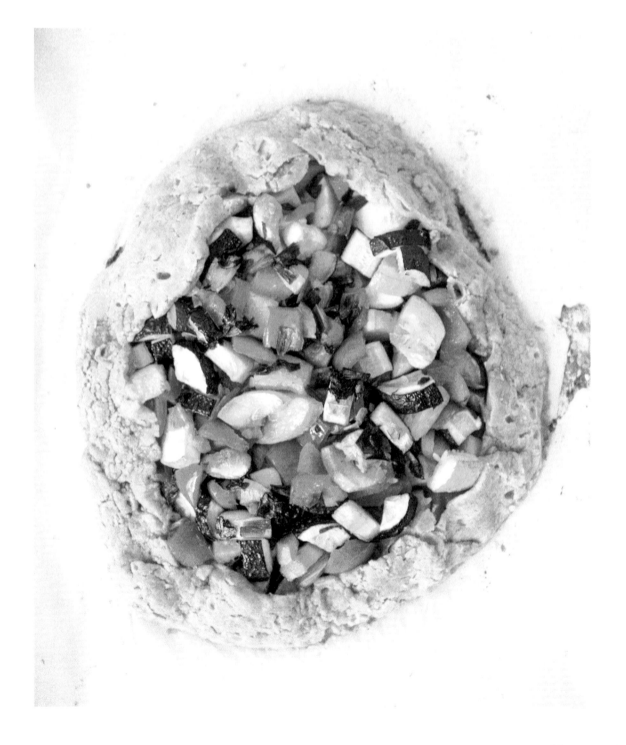

DESSERTS

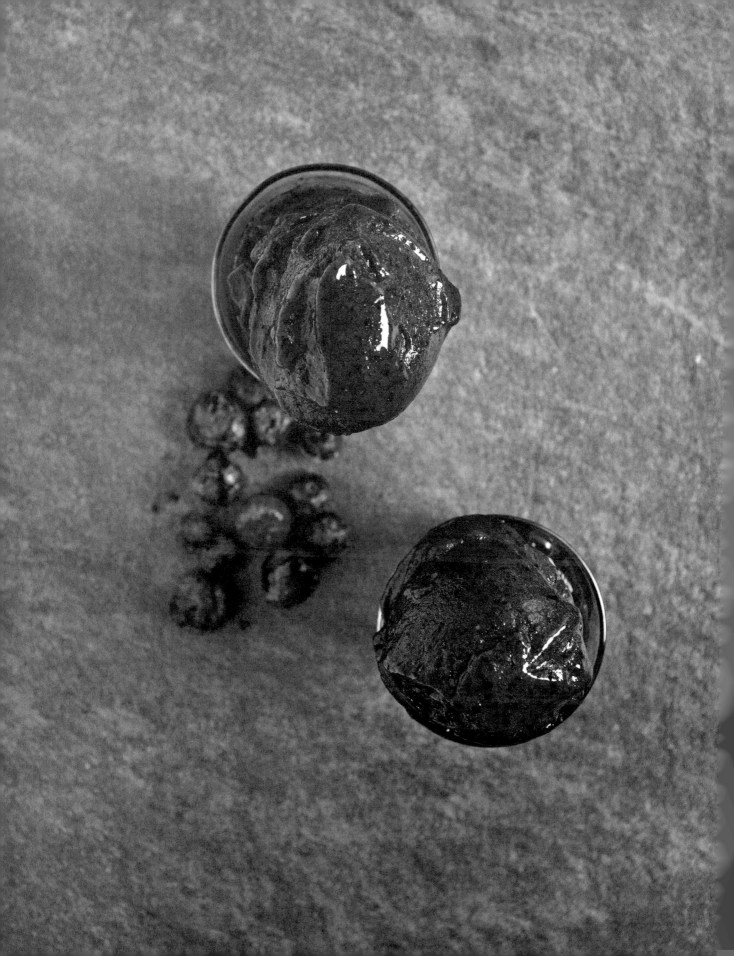

Cherry Berry Sorbet

A healthy frozen treat in a flash! Using frozen fruit makes this recipe super-fast to whip up, and it's high in antioxidants and inflammation-fighting flavonoids—so it's good for you. Eat this when you're craving ice cream but want something low-cal, low-fat, and dairy-free. The syrup or honey offsets the bitterness of the tart cherries.

····· FAST · KID FRIENDLY · LOW CAL · SUPERFOOD · VEGAN ·····
PREP TIME: 5 minutes • TOTAL TIME: 5 minutes

1 cup frozen cherries
1 cup frozen blueberries
1 tablespoon maple syrup or
  pasteurized honey

In the bowl of a food processor, add the cherries, blueberries, and maple syrup or honey and blend until smooth.

Note

Use half tart cherries and half Bing for sweetness. Tart cherries have higher concentrations of anti-inflammatory phytonutrients than sweet cherries. Studies have shown that they reduce pain, inflammation, and gout, improve sleep, and can decrease muscle soreness from exercise. Most grocery stores carry frozen blends.

Variation

You can use pretty much any frozen fruit into a sorbet. Mangos, in particular, will help thicken other fruit blends. If your sorbet becomes too thick, add a little water to the food processor to help smooth it out a little bit.

Shortbread Cookies

These tasty treats have really simple ingredients, so they're easy to make at home. The maple sugar adds a nice warmth to the flavor, and it has a lower glycemic index than regular sugar, so your blood-sugar levels won't roller-coaster after you eat these.

····· CROWD PLEASER · KID FRIENDLY · VEGETARIAN ·····

PREP TIME: 15 minutes • COOK TIME: 15 minutes • TOTAL TIME: 30 minutes

1 cup butter

½ cup powdered maple sugar or coconut sugar

2 cups All-Purpose Flour Blend (page 28)

½ teaspoon xanthan gum

1 egg

1 teaspoon vanilla extract

1 pinch salt

1. Preheat the oven to 350°F.

2. Line a baking sheet with parchment paper.

3. In the bowl of a stand mixer, cream the butter and sugar.

4. Add the All-Purpose Flour Blend, xanthan gum, and salt. Mix well until they combine.

5. On a large cutting board dusted with some All-Purpose Flour Blend, roll out the dough to a ⅓-inch thickness.

6. Cut the dough into the shapes of your choice.

7. Lay the cookies on the prepared baking sheet, leaving 1 inch among all cookies.

8. Bake for 15 minutes or until golden.

Tip

To make the powdered sugar, pulse ½ cup maple sugar or coconut sugar in a food processor into a powder.

Variation

To make this vegan, omit the egg and xanthan gum and add 1 tablespoon ground chia seeds mixed with 2–3 tablespoons water to create the dough.

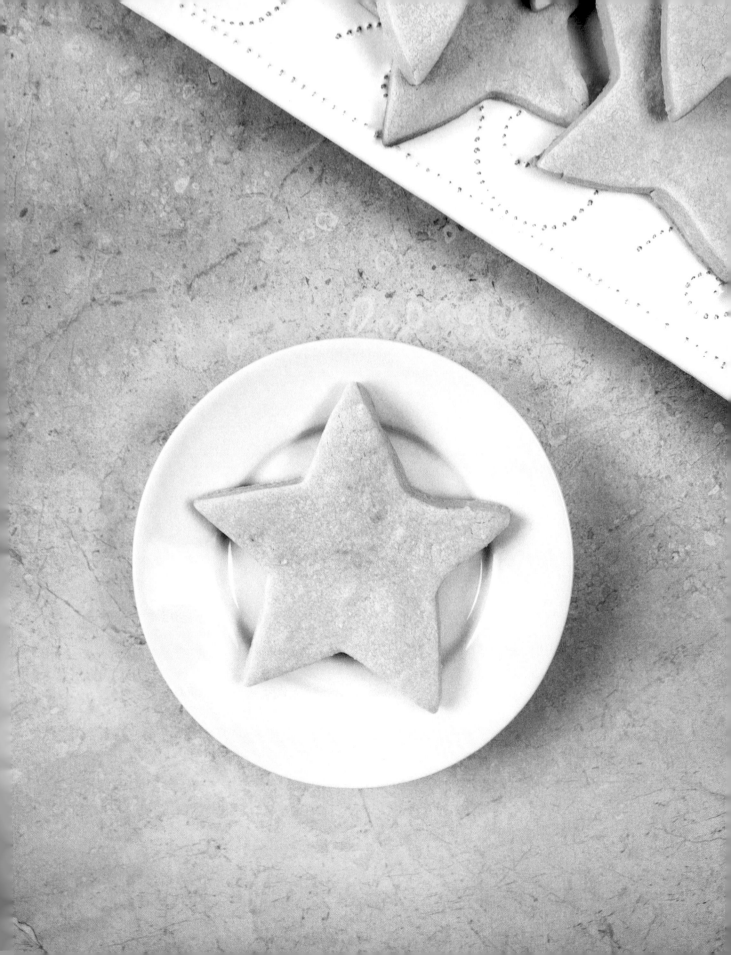

Carrot Apple Cupcakes

You should add fruits or vegetables to everything you eat in order to consume more nutrients and antioxidants. These lovely little cupcakes are no exception—and, better yet, they include both fruits *and* veggies! They taste light and fluffy, but they provide loads of vitamins A and C and quercetin, our mast-stabilizing superstar. The water content of the carrots and apples keep the cupcakes nice and naturally moist.

····· CROWD PLEASER · DAIRY FREE · KID FRIENDLY · VEGETARIAN ·····
PREP TIME: 30 minutes · COOK TIME: 20 minutes · TOTAL TIME: 50 minutes

3 yellow or orange carrots
(to yield 1½ cups)
2 red apples (to yield 1 cup)
1 teaspoon vanilla extract
4 eggs
1 cup extra-light olive oil
2 cups All-Purpose Flour
Blend (page 28)
1 cup sugar or coconut sugar
2 teaspoons baking powder
¼ teaspoon salt
½ cup milk of choice
freeze-dried apple chunks
for garnish

FROSTING

3 (13½-ounce) cans coconut
cream (refrigerated for
24 hours)
2 tablespoons maple syrup
or pasteurized honey
1 teaspoon vanilla extract

1. Preheat the oven to 350°F.

2. Peel and shred the carrots and peel and core apples. In a food processor, puree both.

3. Prepare 2 (12-count) muffin tins with parchment liners or greasing the cavities with a little extra-light olive oil.

4. In a large mixing bowl, combine the carrot and apple puree, vanilla extract, eggs, and olive oil and mix together.

5. In a separate bowl, combine the All-Puprose Flour Blend, sugar, baking powder, and salt.

6. Add the dry ingredients to wet ingredients, alternating with the milk until a moist batter forms.

7. Divide the batter evenly in the muffin tins—up to the top if you want because gluten-free cupcakes don't rise as much—and bake for 20 minutes or until a toothpick inserted into the middle of a cupcake comes out clean.

8. Let cool completely, about 30 minutes, before frosting.

9. In the bowl of a stand mixer, add the coconut cream solids—being careful to avoid using any liquid—maple syrup or honey, and vanilla extract and whip until thick, about 5 minutes.

10. Frost the cupcakes, garnish with freeze-dried apple chunks, then refrigerate them to keep the frosting nice and firm.

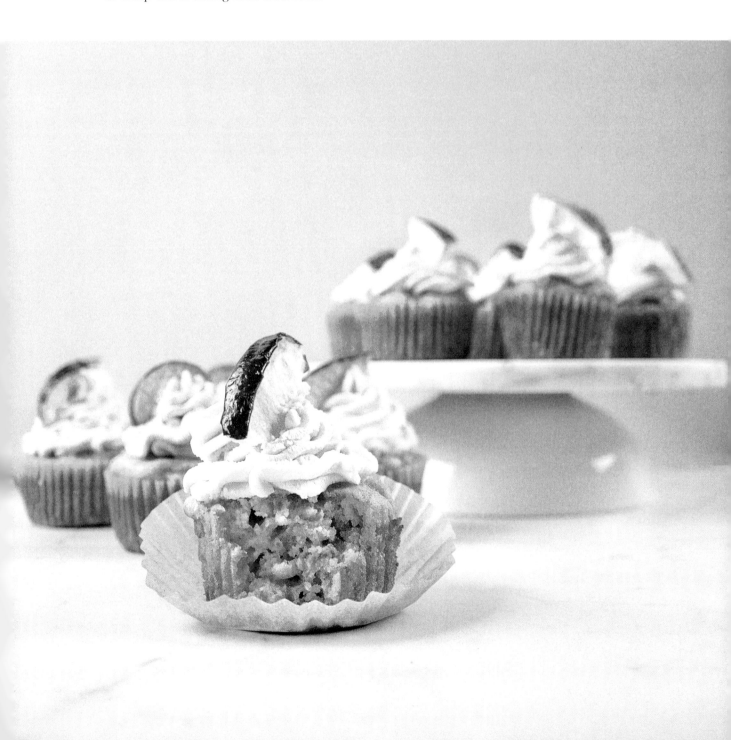

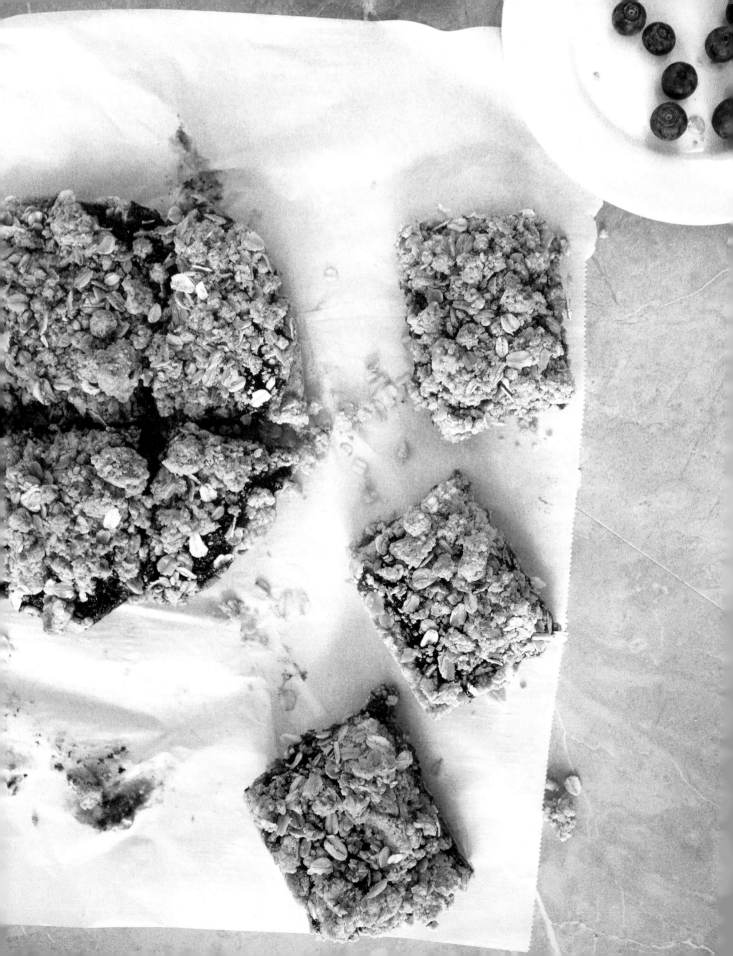

Blueberry Bars

These yummy bars work equally well as snacks or as dessert. They also freeze well for bringing on road trips or hikes. The coconut oil increases the anti-inflammatory power of the bars, and coconut sugar is kinder on your system than regular sugar.

····· GREAT SNACK · KID FRIENDLY · LOW FODMAP · VEGAN ·····

PREP TIME: 35 minutes • COOK TIME: 15 minutes • TOTAL TIME: 50 minutes

½ cup coconut oil

⅓ cup + ½ cup rolled oats

1½ cups All-Purpose Flour Blend (page 28)

⅔ cup brown sugar or coconut sugar

1 teaspoon vanilla extract

1 teaspoon baking powder

¼ cup water

FILLING

3 cups frozen blueberries

¼ cup maple syrup

2 tablespoons tapioca starch

1 teaspoon vanilla extract

1. Preheat the oven to 375°F.

2. In a food processor, pulse 1⅓ cups of rolled oats into 1 cup of oat flour.

3. In the bowl of a stand mixer, combine the coconut oil, oat flour, All-Purpose Flour Blend, sugar, vanilla extract, baking powder, and water.

4. Divide the mixture and press half of it into the bottom of an 8 x 8-inch baking pan.

5. Next, make the filling. In a medium saucepan over medium heat, cook the blueberries, maple syrup, tapioca starch, and vanilla extract for about 10 minutes, stirring every 3–4 minutes, until it bubbles and thickens.

6. Layer the blueberry filling over the oatmeal batter in the baking pan.

7. Into the remaining oat mixture, add the remaining ½ cup of oats and combine with your fingers.

8. Spread the oat clumps over the blueberry filling.

9. Bake for about 30 minutes, until the oat clumps turn golden.

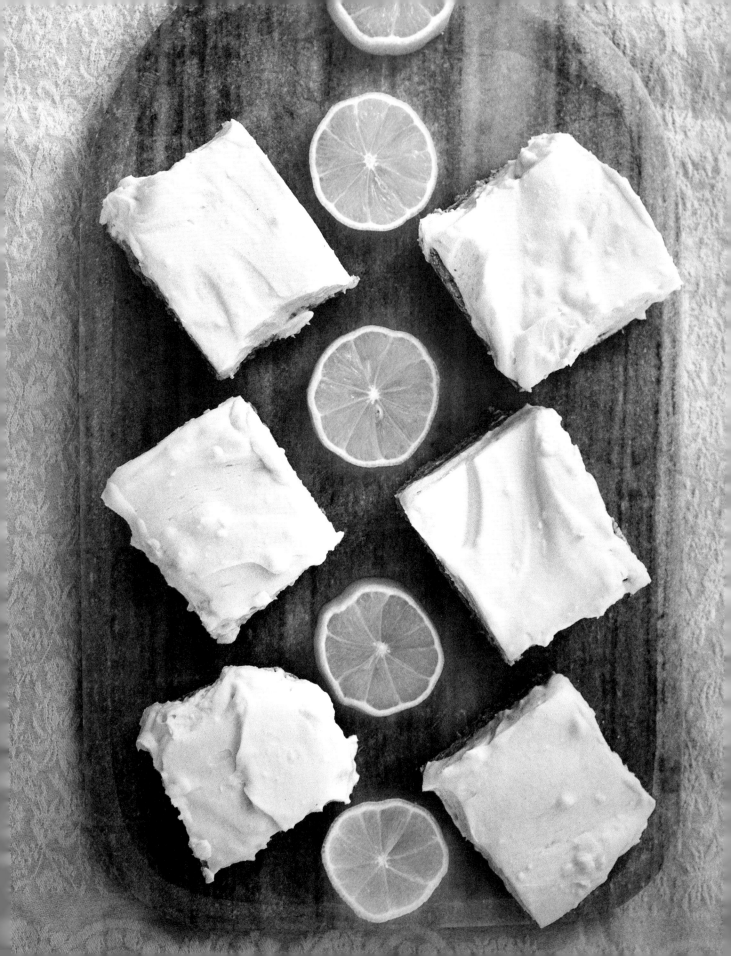

Coconut Lemon Bars

These light and creamy bars have very little lemon flavor in them in order to keep histamine levels low. Sweetened only lightly with a little maple syrup or honey, they also have low levels of natural sugars. The whole-grain crust provides lots of fiber, though, so these are a great healthy option for a party or picnic.

····· CROWD PLEASER · VEGAN ·····

PREP TIME: 45 minutes • COOK TIME: 15 minutes • TOTAL TIME: 1 hour

CRUST

1½ cups rolled oats
¼ cup shredded unsulfured, unsweetened coconut
½ cup coconut oil
1 tablespoon maple syrup or pasteurized honey
½ cup All-Purpose Flour Blend (page 28)

FROSTING

2 (13½-ounce) cans coconut cream (refrigerated for 24 hours)
juice of 1 lemon
3 tablespoons maple syrup or pasteurized honey

1. Preheat the oven to 350°F.

2. First, make the crust. In a food processor, grind the oats and coconut together.

3. Add the coconut oil, maple syrup or honey, and All-Puporse Flour Blend and pulse until the batter forms a ball.

4. Press the crust into an 8 x 8-inch square baking dish.

5. Bake the crust for 12–15 minutes or until lightly golden. Let cool completely, about 30 minutes.

6. Next, make the filling. In the bowl of a stand mixer fitted with the paddle attachment, add the coconut cream solids—making sure not to add any liquid from the can—lemon juice, and maple syrup or honey. Whip until fluffy, about 5 minutes.

7. Spread the filling onto the crust and refrigerate for at least 1 hour.

8. When ready to serve, cut into 12 bars.

> ### Variation
> *Peppermint and lemon complement each other nicely, so add some fresh peppermint to the cream filling. Mince the leaves of 1 handful of fresh peppermint and add while whipping the cream.*

Blueberry Peach Galette

This open-faced pie is another crowd favorite that's great for impressing loved ones at dinner parties. The fruit as the base makes this dessert healthier, and the sugar adds a nice crunch to the crust. This recipe is much faster to make than a normal pie because you leave it looking rough around the edges and it cooks faster because it's open-faced.

····· CROWD PLEASER · KID FRIENDLY · VEGAN ·····

PREP TIME: 50 minutes · COOK TIME: 40 minutes · TOTAL TIME: 1 hour 30 minutes

DOUGH

⅔ cup rolled oats

2 cups All-Purpose Flour Blend (page 28)

1 tablespoon sugar or coconut sugar

½ teaspoon salt

1½ cups unsalted butter or coconut oil

⅔ cup ice water

FILLING

3 cups frozen wild blueberries, defrosted

1 cup fresh peaches in ¼-inch slices

2 tablespoons tapioca starch

¼ cup turbinado sugar or coconut sugar

1 pinch salt

TOPPING

1 tablespoon milk of choice

1 tablespoon turbinado sugar

1. First, make the dough.

2. In a food processor, pulse the rolled oats into ½ cup of oat flour.

3. In a large bowl, combine the dry ingredients.

4. In 1 tablespoon portions, add the butter or coconut oil to the bowl. If using butter, use a pastry blender to cut the butter into the dry ingredients until it forms pea-size lumps.

5. Slowly add the ice water and mix until the ingredients just combine and form a dough. Add more water if necessary to bring the dough together.

6. Form the dough into a ball, cover it in plastic wrap, and refrigerate it for at least 30 minutes or overnight.

7. Preheat the oven to 375°F.

8. On a surface dusted with some All-Purpose Flour Blend, roll out the dough to a ⅓-inch thickness and then place it onto a cookie sheet.

9. In a medium saucepan over medium-low heat, cook the blueberries, peaches, tapioca starch, sugar, and salt for about 7 minutes or until the peaches just become tender.

10. Pour the cooked fruit in the center of the tart crust, leaving a 3-inch border.

11. Fold the crust over the edge of the fruit and seal any holes.

12. Brush the crust with the milk and sprinkle with the turbinado sugar crystals.

13. Bake for 40 minutes or until the base of the tart turns golden.

14. Serve a la carte or top with Whipped Coconut Cream (page 63).

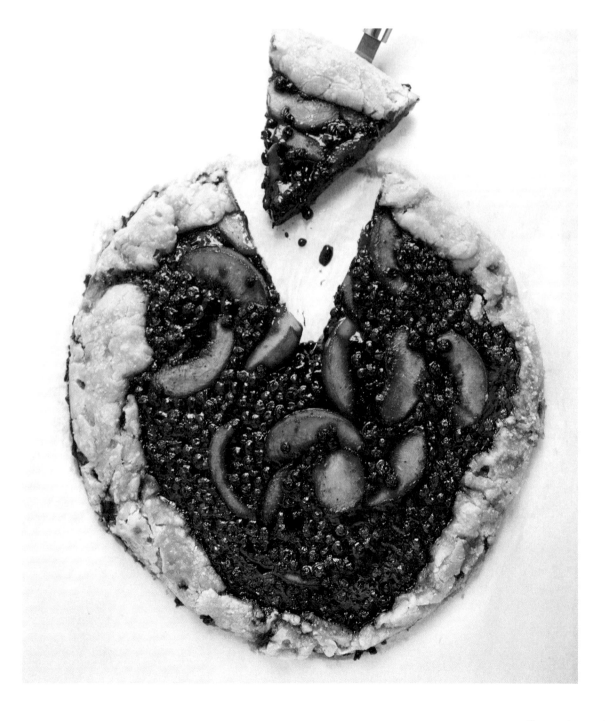

Fruit Tart with Mascarpone Cream

This is my all-time favorite dessert. I've had it for my birthday—instead of birthday cake—for the last three years. The creaminess of the filling tastes just lovely with this crust, and the fruit provides a nice, bright contrast along with healthy antioxidants. Mascarpone tastes amazing, but you can use Whipped Coconut Cream for a vegan version (see the Variation). I like to use oats in all of my baked recipes because they make the gluten-free flours taste more like wheat and add more fiber.

····· CROWD PLEASER · KID FRIENDLY · VEGETARIAN ·····

PREP TIME: 1 hour 10 minutes · COOK TIME: 20 minutes · TOTAL TIME: 1 hour 30 minutes

DOUGH

⅓ cup rolled oats

1¼ cups All-Purpose Flour Blend (page 28)

1 tablespoon coconut sugar or regular sugar

½ teaspoon salt

1 cup unsalted butter

⅔ cup ice water

FILLING

1 cup cold whipping cream

8 ounces mascarpone cheese

½ cup confectioners' sugar or powdered coconut sugar (processed from ½ cup regular sugar)

1 teaspoon vanilla extract

1 pint blueberries or fruit of choice

1. First, make the dough.

2. In a food processor, pulse the rolled oats into ¼ cup of oat flour.

3. In the bowl of a stand mixer, combine the flours, sugar, and salt.

4. In 1 tablespoon portions, add the butter to the bowl and use a pastry blender to cut the butter into the dry ingredients until they form pea-size lumps.

5. Slowly add the ice water and mix until the ingredients just combine and form a dough.

6. Form the dough into a ball, cover it in plastic wrap, and refrigerate it for at least 30 minutes or overnight.

7. Preheat oven to 375°F.

8. On a large sheet of parchment paper, place dough then top with another sheet of parchment paper. Roll out the dough between the sheets of parchment paper until ¼-inch thick.

9. Place the dough into a 9-inch tart pan and make fork holes in it so air can escape as it bakes.

10. Bake the crust for 15–20 minutes or until it turns golden brown. Let it cool completely, about 30 minutes.

11. In the bowl of a stand mixer, add the whipping cream and, with the whisk attachment, whisk until soft peaks form.

12. Add the mascarpone cheese, sugar, and vanilla extract and whisk until just combined, about 30 seconds.

11. Add the cream filling to the cooled tart shell, then layer the fruit on top.

12. Chill until ready to serve.

Variation

To make this vegan, substitute 1 cup coconut oil for the butter in the crust, and for the filling use Whipped Coconut Cream (page 63).

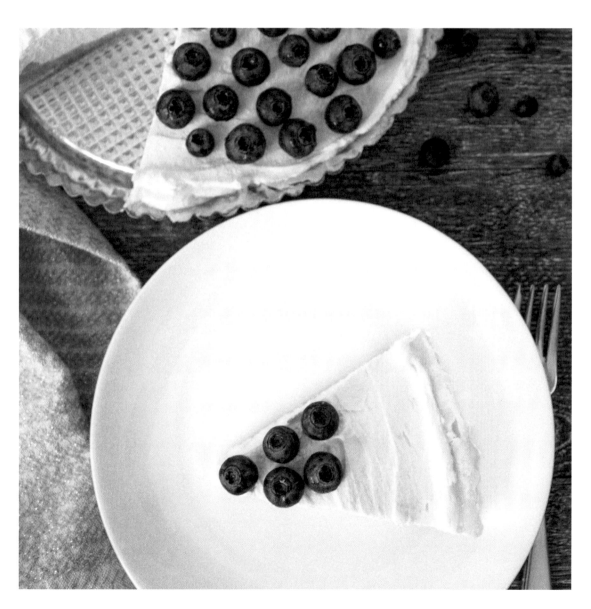

Mango Cantaloupe Sorbet

You can find frozen mango chunks at most grocery stores these days, but you'll have to freeze your own cantaloupe chunks in advance. It's worth it, though, because this sorbet is rich in vitamin C, making it a great immune-system booster and a powerful anti-inflammatory dessert that's perfect for the dog days of summer.

····· KID FRIENDLY · LOW CAL · SUPERFOOD · VEGAN ·····

PREP TIME: **2 hours 10 minutes** • TOTAL TIME: **2 hours 10 minutes**

¼ cantaloupe
1 cup frozen mango chunks

1. Cut the cantaloupe into ⅓-inch chunks and freeze for at least 2 hours.

2. In the bowl of a food processor, add frozen fruit chunks.

3. Blend until smooth, adding a little water if necessary.

> **Variation**
>
> *If you don't want to wait for the cantaloupe to freeze, use frozen peaches instead, which you can find at most grocery stores.*
>
> *Add 4 tablespoons heavy cream to make this dish taste creamier and more indulgent.*

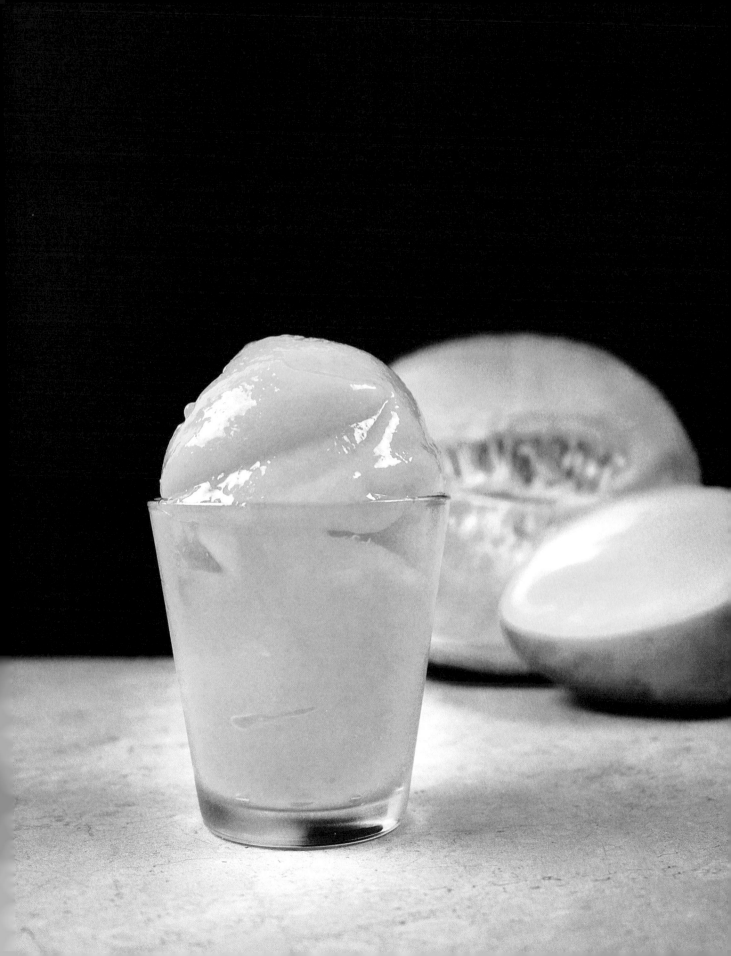

SAUCES & CONDIMENTS

Applesauce

Serve this simple, easy dish with the Zucchini Latkes (page 184) or have it on its own as a light and healthy snack.

····· FAST · GREAT SNACK · KID FRIENDLY · LOW CAL · VEGAN ·····
PREP TIME: 10 minutes • COOK TIME: 15 minutes • TOTAL TIME: 25 minutes

3 red apples
¼ cup water
maple syrup (optional)

1. Peel, core, and chop the apples.

2. In a medium saucepan over medium heat, add the apples and water and cook for about 15 minutes, or until the apples have softened.

3. Use a potato masher or immersion blender to mash or puree the apples to the preferred consistency.

4. If the applesauce tastes too tart, add a drizzle of maple syrup to sweeten it.

Basil Dressing

This summery, herbaceous dressing tastes phenomenal on salad, fish, or chicken. Try it on the Salmon & Vegetable Medley (page 155) or the Grilled Chicken & Vegetables (page 156). Feel free to add or substitute other herbs, such as dill, oregano, parsley, rosemary, or sage.

····· FAST · SUPERFOOD · VEGAN ·····

PREP TIME: **10** minutes • TOTAL TIME: **10** minutes

1 clove garlic

½ cup fresh basil leaves

juice of 1 lemon

½ cup extra-virgin olive oil

½ teaspoon salt

In a blender or food processor, combine the garlic, basil, lemon juice, olive oil, and salt and blend until smooth.

> **Tip**
>
> *If you can't handle the garlic raw, sauté the clove in a little olive oil for a few minutes to soften it before blending, use garlic-infused oil, or let the clove steep in the oil and remove it before blending.*

Blueberry Jam

This delicious, anti-inflammatory jam tastes amazing with the Maple Stovetop Donuts (page 39), Soft Oatmeal Bread (page 58), and Shortbread Cookies (page 208), and you can make this simple jam with other low-histamine fruits as well.

····· LOW FODMAP · SUPERFOOD · VEGAN ·····
PREP TIME: 5 minutes • COOK TIME: 15 minutes • TOTAL TIME: 20 minutes

2 cups frozen wild
  blueberries
2 tablespoons tapioca starch
¼ cup maple syrup or
  coconut sugar

1. In a small saucepan over medium-low heat, cook all ingredients for about 15 minutes or until bubbly, stirring occasionally.

2. When the jam starts to thicken, remove from heat and let cool.

Caesar Dressing

Mascarpone cheese gives this dressing a creamy taste, and the lemon and garlic add lots of tang. Unlike the real thing, this version is vegetarian—no fish! Try it with the Super Salad (page 86) or as a dip for the Thyme Garlic Fries (page 145).

····· FAST · VEGETARIAN ·····
PREP TIME: 10 minutes • TOTAL TIME: 10 minutes

1 clove garlic
¼ cup extra-virgin olive oil
juice of 1 lemon
½ teaspoon salt
¼ cup mascarpone cheese

In a blender, combine the garlic, olive oil, lemon juice, salt, and mascarpone and blend until smooth.

Tip

If you can't tolerate raw garlic, sauté the clove in olive oil for a few minutes to soften it before blending, or let the clove steep in the oil and remove it before blending.

Caramelized Onions

Slow cooking enhances the sweetness of the onions, which deliciously enhance the White Bean & Basil Cakes (page 120), Arugula Pizza (page 191), Black Bean Burgers (page 160), and Lettuce-Wrapped Burgers (page 167).

····· CROWD PLEASER · LOW CAL · SUPERFOOD · VEGAN ·····

PREP TIME: 10 minutes • COOK TIME: 12 hours • TOTAL TIME: 12 hours 10 minutes

3 pounds sweet onions

2 tablespoons extra-virgin olive oil

½ teaspoon salt

1. Cut the onions into ¼-inch slices and add them to a slow cooker with the olive oil and salt.

2. Cook on low for 10–12 hours.

VARIATION WHITOUT SLOW COOKER

If you don't have a slow cooker or don't have 12 hours to make this recipe, here's the stovetop version.

PREP TIME: 10 minutes • COOK TIME: 1 hour • TOTAL TIME: 1 hour 10 minutes

2 large sweet onions

¼ cup water

1 tablespoon extra-virgin olive oil

½ teaspoon salt

1. Cut the onions into ¼-inch slices.

2. In a medium pan over medium heat, combine the onions, water, olive oil, and salt. Cover, reduce heat to medium-low, and simmer for about 1 hour or until the onions caramelize and become very tender.

> **Tip**
> *Freeze extra onions in ice cube trays for up to 3 months.*

Cranberry Chutney

This chutney is easy enough for a weeknight meal but makes a great addition to your Thanksgiving spread. Try it with the Lettuce-Wrapped Burgers (page 167) or Rosemary & Garlic Chicken Breasts with Vegetables (page 200).

····· SUPERFOOD · VEGAN ·····

PREP TIME: 15 minutes • COOK TIME: 15 minutes • TOTAL TIME: 30 minutes

1 tablespoon finely grated
   fresh ginger
1 red apple
2 shallots
12 ounces fresh cranberries
1 tablespoon extra-light
   olive oil
1 cup sugar or coconut sugar
½ teaspoon salt
1 cup water

1. Prepare the ginger; peel, core, and dice the apple; mince the shallots; and rinse the cranberries.

2. In a large saucepan over medium-low heat, add the shallots, ginger, and oil and cook about 5 minutes or until the shallots soften.

3. Add the apple, cranberries, sugar, salt, and water.

4. Bring to a boil, then reduce to a simmer, stirring occasionally, for about 10–15 minutes or until most of the berries have burst and the sauce is starting to thicken.

5. Remove from heat and cool in the refrigerator completely before serving.

Garlic Croutons

Here's an easy way to make yummy croutons from the Soft Oatmeal Bread on page 58.

····· DAIRY FREE · KID FRIENDLY · LOW FODMAP · VEGETARIAN ·····

PREP TIME: 10 minutes • COOK TIME: 10 minutes • TOTAL TIME: 20 minutes

2 large slices Soft Oatmeal Bread (page 58)

½ teaspoon salt

1 clove garlic

1 tablespoon fresh parsley

1 tablespoon fresh rosemary

3 tablespoons extra-light olive oil

1. Preheat oven to 400°F and line a baking sheet with parchment paper.

2. Cut the bread into 1-inch pieces and set aside.

3. In a food processor, pulse the salt, garlic, parsley, rosemary, and olive oil and then toss with the bread.

4. Bake the croutons for about 10 minutes or until golden brown.

Ketchup

The ratio of onions to tomato makes this low-histamine recipe a great alternative to the store-bought condiment. Histamine increases in tomatoes as they ripen, so chose yellow or unripe red tomatoes. Enjoy this on the Black Bean Burgers (page 160), Lettuce-Wrapped Burgers (page 167), and Thyme Garlic Fries (page 145).

····· CROWD PLEASER · KID FRIENDLY · LOW CAL · VEGAN ·····

PREP TIME: 15 minutes • COOK TIME: 30 minutes • TOTAL TIME: 45 minutes

1 yellow or under-ripe red tomato

2 large sweet onions

1 clove garlic

¼ cup sugar or coconut sugar

1 teaspoon salt

¼ cup water

1 tablespoon extra-light olive oil

1. Dice the tomato and onions.

2. In a medium saucepan, simmer all ingredients for about 30 minutes or until the onions have become tender.

3. With an immersion blender, blend all ingredients until smooth.

Mango Salsa

This lovely, summery salsa is tomato-free but full of flavor. Enjoy it on the Mango Salsa Salmon (page 148) or as a dip with chips made from the Corn Tortillas (page 101).

····· FAST · LOW CAL · VEGAN ·····

PREP TIME: 10 minutes • TOTAL TIME: 10 minutes

1 mango
½ red bell pepper
2 tablespoons chopped
   scallions
1 teaspoon lime juice
1 teaspoon extra-light
   olive oil
salt

1. Pit, peel, and dice the mango and dice the bell pepper.

2. In a bowl, combine the mango, bell pepper, scallions, lime juice, olive oil, and salt to taste.

Mango Sauce

This quick sauce creates the ultimate flavor boost to any meal. Enjoy it on the Cod Cakes or drizzled over the Grilled Chicken & Vegetables (page 156).

····· CROWD PLEASER · FAST · LOW CAL · VEGAN ·····

PREP TIME: 5 minutes • COOK TIME: 10 minutes • TOTAL TIME: 15 minutes

1 cup frozen or fresh mango, chopped

¼ cup chopped red, orange, or yellow bell pepper

2 scallions

¼ cup water

2 tablespoons extra-light olive oil

1. Prepare the mango and bell pepper and chop the scallions.

2. In a small pot over medium heat, simmer all ingredients for 5–10 minutes, until the vegetables become tender.

3. Transfer ingredients to a blender and blend until smooth.

Tip

You can freeze the sauce in ice cube trays for up to 3 months.

No-mato Pomodoro Sauce

If tomatoes bother you, you're going to love this sauce. Pour it over the Spaghetti Squash Pasta with Chicken Meatballs (page 192) or use it as a pasta or pizza sauce.

····· LOW CAL · SUPERFOOD · VEGAN ·····

PREP TIME: 5 minutes • COOK TIME: 20 minutes • TOTAL TIME: 25 minutes

2 cups chopped fresh basil

2 red bell peppers

2 cloves garlic

2 sweet onions

2 tablespoons extra-virgin olive oil

¼ cup water

1. Prepare the basil, small-dice the bell peppers, mince the garlic, and dice the onions.

2. In a medium pot over medium heat, add the bell peppers, garlic, onions, olive oil, and water. Simmer for 15 minutes or until the vegetables become tender.

3. Add the basil and cook for another 5 minutes.

Pomodoro Sauce

If tomatoes don't bother your stomach, this is the sauce you want. Pour it over the Spaghetti Squash Pasta with Chicken Meatballs (page 192) or use it as a pasta or pizza sauce.

····· LOW CAL · VEGAN ·····

PREP TIME: 10 minutes · COOK TIME: 35 minutes · TOTAL TIME: 45 minutes

1 cup chopped fresh basil

2 medium tomatoes

2 cloves garlic

2 large sweet onions

2 tablespoons extra-virgin olive oil

1 tablespoon dried oregano

salt

1. Prepare the basil, chop the tomatoes, mince the garlic, and dice the onions.

2. In a medium pan over medium heat, sauté the onions and garlic in the olive oil for 2–3 minutes.

3. Add the chopped tomatoes, oregano, and salt to taste and simmer for about 30 minutes or until the pieces of tomato break down and the onions have become tender.

4. Add the basil and continue simmering for 1 minute.

> **Tip**
>
> *Freeze extra sauce in ice cube trays for up to 3 months.*

Ranch Dressing

This low-histamine dressing has no added preservatives or flavoring agents, but you can freeze it for up to 3 months and thaw whenever you like. Try it in the Cauliflower Mash (page 133) instead of the garlic, broth, and butter; on the Super Salad (page 86); or on a simple garden salad.

CROWD PLEASER · FAST · KID FRIENDLY · VEGETARIAN

PREP TIME: 10 minutes · TOTAL TIME: 10 minutes

1 ounce cream cheese or
   mascarpone cheese
¼ cup chopped fresh dill
½ clove garlic
2 tablespoons chopped fresh
   chives
¼ cup milk of choice
salt
¼ cup extra-virgin olive oil

In a blender, combine all ingredients and blend until smooth.

Sesame Garlic Dressing

Enjoy this bright, nutty, balanced dressing on the Super Salad (page 86) or the Fall Harvest Salad (page 129).

······ FAST · VEGAN ······

PREP TIME: 10 minutes · TOTAL TIME: 10 minutes

4 tablespoons sesame seeds

juice of 1 lemon

1 clove garlic

½ cup extra-virgin olive oil

1 pinch salt

In a blender or food processor, combine all ingredients and blend until smooth.

Tip

If raw garlic bothers your stomach, sauté it in olive oil for 2–3 minutes before blending the dressing or let the clove steep in the olive oil for 20 minutes and remove before it before blending.

Vegan Pesto

This pesto is a great way to sneak some extra greens into your diet. Enjoy it on the Pesto Penne with Asparagus (page 151) or as a spread for a veggie sandwich.

····· FAST · HIGH PROTEIN · SUPERFOOD · VEGAN ·····

PREP TIME: 15 minutes • TOTAL TIME: 15 minutes

1 bunch stinging nettles
   (optional)
2 large Swiss chard leaves
2 cups chopped fresh basil
   leaves
¼ cup raw pumpkin seeds
¼ cup extra-virgin olive oil
juice of ½ lemon
1 clove garlic

1. If using stinging nettles, bring a medium pot full of water to a boil, add nettles, and blanch for 1 minute. Remove from the pot, remove the leaves from the stems, discard the stems, and add the leaves to the pesto ingredients.

2. Remove the stems and central veins of the Swiss chard and prepare the basil.

3. In a food processor, combine all ingredients and blend until smooth. Add a little water if the mixture is too thick.

Variation

To make this recipe low FODMAP, steep the clove of garlic in olive oil for 10–20 minutes and remove before blending.

Vegetable Broth

Keep single or double servings of this super handy staple in your freezer for quick use in the Kale & White Bean Soup (page 115), Superfood Stew (page 119), Cauliflower Mash (page 133), Mushroom Risotto (page 186), and other recipes. Also feel free to add your favorite herbs, spices, and veggies to the mix.

····· LOW CAL · SUPERFOOD · VEGAN ·····

PREP TIME: 20 minutes • COOK TIME: 2 hours 30 minutes • TOTAL TIME: 2 hours 50 minutes

1 sweet potato

1 potato

2 large sweet onions

4 cremini mushrooms

9 cups water

2 stalks celery

3 carrots

2 bay leaves

1 handful fresh parsley leaves

1 handful fresh thyme sprigs, including stems

2 teaspoons salt

1. Quarter the potatoes and onions and rinse the mushrooms.

2. In a large pot, add all ingredients and heat to a boil.

3. Reduce heat to medium-low and simmer for 2½ hours.

4. Remove the herbs and vegetables.

Tip

Freeze the broth in 1-cup servings for up to 3 months.

At-a-Glance Recipe Table

	RECIPE	CROWD PLEASER	DAIRY FREE	FAST	GREAT SNACK	HIGH PROTEIN	KID FRIENDLY
BREAKFAST	All-Purpose Flour Blend			●			
	Apple Oatmeal Bars	●	●		●		●
	Blueberries & Cream Smoothie Bowl			●		●	●
	Blueberry Corn Muffins		●		●		●
	Coconut Crunch Granola				●		
	Coconut Forbidden Rice Pudding						
	Cornmeal Waffle Egg Sandwiches	●					
	Crepes with Blueberries & Whipped Cream	●					
	Maple Scones	●			●		●
	Maple Stovetop Donuts	●			●		●
	Oat Pancakes with Apple Compote		●				●
	Oatmeal Rolls		●				●
	Purple Sweet Potato Donuts	●	●		●		●
	Quick Oats with Berries, Chia & Maple Syrup			●			
	Soft Ginger Granola				●		●
	Soft Oatmeal Bread		●				
	Sweet Potato Ginger Muffins		●		●		
	Sweet Potato Hash with Fried Eggs	●				●	
	Vegetable Omelet					●	
SNACKS	Deep Purple Smoothie			●	●		●
	Fruit Plate with Whipped Coconut Cream	●		●	●		
	Herb Popcorn	●		●	●		
	Macadamia Nut Crunch			●	●	●	●
	Mango Coconut Smoothie			●	●		●
	Maple Sugar Popcorn			●	●		●
	Melon Cooler			●	●		●
	Oat Crackers				●		
	Rice Cakes with Coconut Butter & Fruit			●	●		
LUNCH	Acorn Squash Soup				●		
	Beet & Sweet Potato Rösti	●	●		●		
	Beets & Greens Salad						
	Butternut Squash & Arugula Salad				●		
	Carrot, Lentil & Kale Salad						

LOW CAL	LOW FODMAP	SUPERFOOD	VEGAN	VEGETARIAN	PAGE
	●		●		28
		●	●	●	51
	●	●	●		31
	●	●		●	52
		●	●		43
		●	●		61
	●			●	44
	●			●	62
				●	56
	●		●		39
		●		●	41
	●			●	46
		●		●	48
	●	●	●		26
	●	●	●		32
	●			●	58
	●	●		●	54
		●		●	35
		●		●	36
		○	○		67
			○		75
○			○		73
		○	○		79
		○	○		68
			○		72
○			○		76
			○		80
○		○	○		71
●		●	●		111
●		●		●	98
●		●	●		103
●		●	●		112
		●	●		95

RECIPE	CROWD PLEASER	DAIRY FREE	FAST	GREAT SNACK	HIGH PROTEIN	KID FRIENDLY
LUNCH						
Corn Tortillas				●		
Garlic Flatbread				●		
Kale & White Bean Soup				●		
Loaded Greek Salad			●			
Mango Bean Salad	●		●		●	
Oat-Flour Wraps				●	●	
Quinoa, Beet & Corn Salad					●	●
Roasted Asparagus with Fried Eggs & Pea Shoots		●				
Roasted Carrot & Garlic Hummus	●			●	●	
Summer Quinoa Salad	●				●	
Super Salad with Sesame Garlic Dressing				●		
Superfood Stew						
Sweet & Savory Salad						
White Bean & Basil Cakes				●	●	●
White Bean & Basil Dip	●		●	●	●	
SIDES						
Butternut Squash with Brown Butter & Sage	●			●		
Cauliflower Mash	●					●
Cucumber Dill Salad			●			
Fall Harvest Salad			●			
Garlic Broccoli			●			
Maple Thyme Carrots	●			●		●
Onion Rings	●	●		●		●
Roasted Vegetables	●					
Rosemary Sea Salt Brussels Sprouts				●		
Summer Succotash	●					
Thyme Garlic Fries	●			●		●
DINNER						
Asian Stir-Fry Noodles						
Basil & Garlic Salmon with Sautéed Greens		●			●	
Beef Tenderloin with Herb Butter					●	
Black Bean Burgers	●			●	●	
Buddha Bowl with Sunflower Dressing					●	
Caramelized Onion & Arugula Pizza	●					●
Cod Cakes with Mango Sauce		●			●	
Fajita Chicken Rice Bowl	●	●			●	
Ginger Vegetable Fried Rice with Sautéed Bok Choy	●			●		
Grilled Chicken & Vegetables	●	●			●	
Lettuce-Wrapped Burgers	●	●			●	●
Mango Salsa Salmon		●			●	
Mockaroni & Cheese	●					●

LOW CAL	LOW FODMAP	SUPERFOOD	VEGAN	VEGETARIAN	PAGE
			●		101
			●		104
		●	●		115
●		●	●		90
		●	●		89
			●		100
		●	●		106
●		●		●	92
			●		116
		●	●		109
●		●	●		86
●		●	●		119
●		●	●	●	97
			●		120
			●		85
		●		●	141
●		●		●	133
●				●	127
●		●	●		129
●		●	●		124
					134
●			●	●	142
●					138
●		●	●		136
			●		130
		●	●		145
		●	●		171
		●			178
					196
			●		160
		●	●		198
				●	191
		●			177
		●			163
				●	188
					156
					167
					148
				●	172

	CROWD PLEASER	DAIRY FREE	FAST	GREAT SNACK	HIGH PROTEIN	KID FRIENDLY
DINNER						
Mushroom Risotto	●					●
Mushroom Rosemary Chicken	●				●	
Oven-Fried Chicken	●	●			●	●
Pesto Penne with Asparagus	●					●
Rosemary & Garlic Chicken with Vegetables		●			●	
Salmon & Vegetable Medley					●	
Salmon Apple Salad		●			●	
Salmon Cakes with Dill Butter				●	●	
Sesame Chicken	●	●			●	
Spaghetti Alfredo	●					
Spaghetti Squash Pasta with Chicken Meatballs & Pomodoro Sauce		●			●	●
Vegetable Coconut Curry						
Vegetable Tart	●			●		
Zucchini Latkes with Applesauce		●		●		●
Zucchini Noodles & Chicken Scampi		●			●	●
DESSERTS						
Blueberry Bars				●		●
Blueberry Peach Galette	●					●
Carrot Apple Cupcakes	●	●				●
Cherry Berry Sorbet			●			●
Coconut Lemon Bars	●					●
Fruit Tart with Mascarpone Cream	●					●
Mango Cantaloupe Sorbet						●
Shortbread Cookies	●					●
SAUCES & CONDIMENTS						
Applesauce			●	●		●
Basil Dressing			●			
Blueberry Jam						
Caesar Dressing			●			
Caramelized Onions	●					
Cranberry Chutney						
Garlic Croutons		●				●
Ketchup	●					●
Mango Salsa			●			
Mango Sauce	●		●			
No-mato Pomodoro Sauce						
Pomodoro Sauce						
Ranch Dressing	●		●			●
Sesame Garlic Dressing			●			
Vegan Pesto			●		●	
Vegetable Broth						

LOW CAL	LOW FODMAP	SUPERFOOD	VEGAN	VEGETARIAN	PAGE
				●	186
					164
					183
			●		151
		●			200
		●			155
					175
		●			181
		●			194
				●	153
					192
		●	●		168
	●			●	202
				●	184
					159
	●		●		213
			●		216
				●	210
●		●	●		207
			●		215
				●	218
●		●	●		220
				●	208
●			●		224
		●	●		225
	●	●	●		226
				●	226
●		●	●		227
		●	●		228
	●			●	229
●			●		229
●			●		230
●			●		231
●		●	●		232
●			●		233
				●	234
			●		235
		●	●		236
●		●	●		237

15-Minute Meals

You can make the recipes labeled "fast" that appear at the beginning of each chapter and that are noted in the recipe table (pages 348–351). Here are lists of quick, 15-minute meal ideas that combine those with recipes that you can batch, freeze, and thaw for your busiest days. When cooking, make extra beans, rice, quinoa, and veggies and freeze them for later. Use thin-cut chicken or fish, which cooks more quickly than thicker cuts. You also can put fresh fruit and salads together quickly. Easy, breezy!

BREAKFAST

- Blueberries & Cream Smoothie Bowl (page 31)
- Quick Oats with Berries, Chia & Maple Syrup (page 26)
- Vegetable Omelet (page 36)

Freezer grab

- Blueberry Corn Muffins (page 52)
- Coconut Crunch Granola with milk of choice and blueberries (page 43)
- Purple Sweet Potato Donuts (page 48)
- Soft Ginger Granola with milk of choice (page 32)
- Sweet Potato Ginger Muffins (page 54)
- Sweet Potato Hash with Fried Eggs (page 35)

LUNCH

- Cucumber Dill Salad with Garlic Flatbread
  (pages 127, 104)
- Fall Harvest Salad with Oat Crackers
  (pages 129, 80)
- Loaded Greek Salad (page 90)
- Mango Bean Salad with Corn Tortillas
  (pages 89, 101)
- Super Salad with Sesame Garlic Dressing
  (page 86)
- Sweet & Savory Salad (page 97)
- White Bean & Basil Dip, Oat-Flour Wrap or
  rice crackers, sliced veggies
  (pages 85, 100)

DINNER (20-MINUTE MEALS

- Buddha Bowl with Sunflower Dressing
  (using frozen rice and beans) (page 198)
- Fajita Chicken Rice bowl (using frozen rice
  and beans) (page 163)
- Mango Salsa Salmon (page 148)
- Pesto Penne with Asparagus (page 151)
- Spaghetti Alfredo (page 153)

Freezer grab

- Beet & Sweet Potato Rösti with Super Salad
  with Sesame Garlic Dressing
  (pages 98, 86)
- Crepes with Roasted Vegetables and
  Caramelized Onions (pages 62, 138, 227)
- Roasted Vegetables, Caramelized Onions,
  black beans, quinoa or rice
  (pages 138, 227)
- Superfood Stew or Acorn Squash Soup with
  Oat Crackers (pages 119, 111, 80)
- White Bean & Basil Cakes with mixed
  greens (page 120)

Freezer grab

- Black Bean Burger, lettuce wrap, salad of
  choice (page 160)
- Ginger Vegetable Fried Rice with Sautéed
  Bok Choy (page 188)
- Mushroom Risotto with steamed
  vegetables (page 186)
- Vegetable Coconut Curry (page 168)

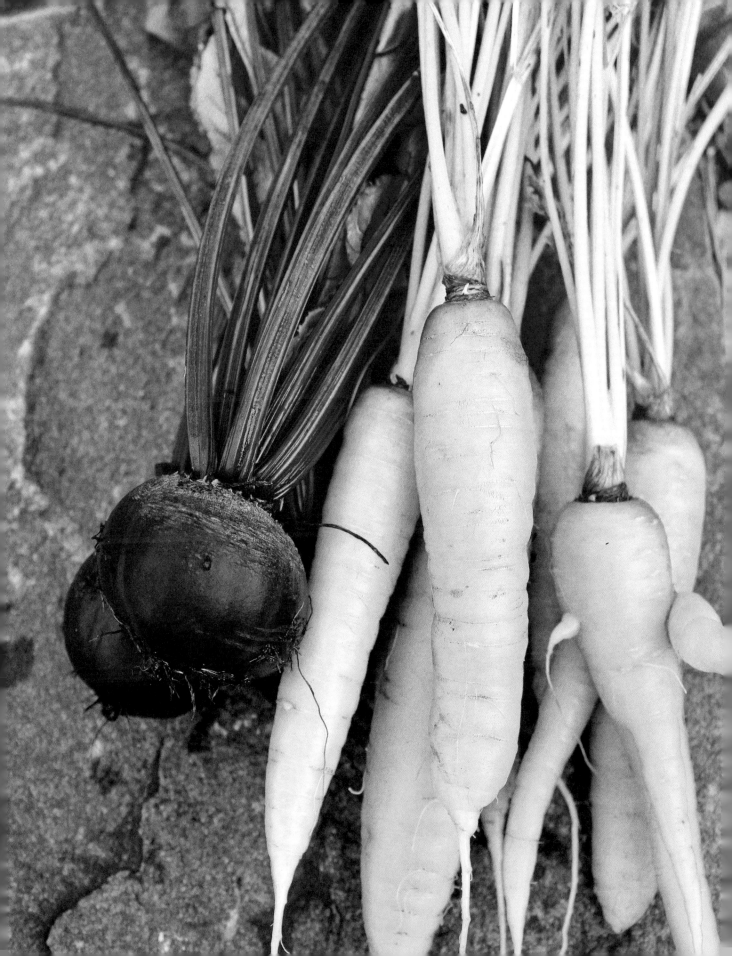

30-Day Meal Plan

....

This meal plan includes repeats on nearby days to save you cooking time. To keep food fresh in the freezer, use good one-quart resealable freezer bags for single portions. When planning portions, make sure that at least half of your plate contains veggies. The plan doesn't indicate portion sizes—since this isn't a calorie-specific or restricted program—but in general one serving of each recipe is a good baseline. If you're still hungry, eat more, but always eat mindfully and slowly and stop eating *before* you feel full.

You can batch and freeze most of the breakfast meals to make life easier. So if you make crepes, muffins, or pancakes on one day, you have breakfast already made for another day. If you don't have time to cook in the morning, a great standby is oatmeal, or eggs with sweet potatoes or veggies. If you can't tolerate chicken eggs, try duck eggs, which tend to cause fewer reactions in people with histamine sensitivity. For salads, it's easy to prep ingredients for three days at a time so you can throw them together the night before. Most of the lunches are vegan or vegetarian so you don't have to worry about histamine creation while your lunch sits in the fridge. The plan includes small amounts of dairy here and there, but you can substitute with nondairy options in many of the recipes. You'll eat lots of whole grains and a moderate amount of nuts and seeds. Eat fish one to two times per week for good omega-3 intake. The plan has low levels of red meat—but it does include a portion or two in the month, and some chicken. Enjoy treats in moderation, two or three times per week—to keep sugar intake low. Drink lots of water every day, along with some healthy teas, coffee if you can handle it, and the occasional pure fruit juice of lower-histamine fruits (page 17).

Feel free to
mix & match
meals—there's
no wrong
way to follow
the plan!

DAY 1

BREAKFAST
Quick Oats with Berries,
Chia & Maple Syrup
(page 26)

SNACK
Fruit Plate with
Whipped Coconut Cream
(page 75)

LUNCH
Acorn Squash Soup,
Garlic Flatbread
(pages 111, 104)

SNACK
Macadamia Nut Crunch,
mango **(page 79)**

DINNER Salmon Cakes
with Dill Butter, mixed
greens, basmati rice
(page 181)

DAY 2

BREAKFAST
Coconut Crunch
Granola, milk of choice,
berries of choice
(page 43)

SNACK
Apple Oatmeal Bar
(page 51)

LUNCH
Roasted Asparagus with
Fried Eggs & Pea Shoots,
fruit of choice **(page 92)**

SNACK
Macadamia Nut Crunch,
grapes **(page 79)**

DINNER
Mango Salsa Salmon
(page 148)

DAY 7

BREAKFAST
Cornmeal Waffle Egg
Sandwiches **(page 44)**

SNACK
Rice Cakes with Coconut
Butter & Fruit **(page 71)**

LUNCH
Quinoa, Beet & Corn
Salad, mixed greens,
fruit of choice **(page 106)**

SNACK
Maple Sugar Popcorn,
apple **(page 72)**

DINNER
Caramelized Onion &
Arugula Pizza, Maple
Thyme Carrots
(pages 191, 134)

DAY 8

BREAKFAST
Coconut Crunch Granola,
milk of choice, berries of
choice **(page 43)**

SNACK
Apple Oatmeal Bar
(page 51)

LUNCH
White Bean & Basil
Cakes, mixed greens,
melon of choice
(page 120)

SNACK
Fruit Plate with
Whipped Coconut Cream
(page 75)

DINNER
Spaghetti Alfredo
(page 153)

DAY 9

BREAKFAST
Quick Oats with Berries,
Chia & Maple Syrup
(page 26)

SNACK
melon of choice,
macadamia nuts

LUNCH
Butternut Squash &
Arugula Salad, Garlic
Flatbread, grapes
(pages 112, 104)

SNACK
Oat Crackers, Whipped
Coconut Cream
(pages 80, 75)

DINNER
Ginger Vegetable Fried
Rice with Sautéed Bok
Choy, Garlic Broccoli
(pages 138, 124)

DAY 10

BREAKFAST
Soft Ginger Granola,
milk of choice **(page 32)**

SNACK
Roasted Carrot & Garlic
Hummus, sliced veggies
of choice **(page 116)**

LUNCH
Fall Harvest Salad,
Oatmeal Roll
(pages 129, 46)

SNACK
Macadamia Nut Crunch,
grapes **(page 79)**

DINNER
Basil & Garlic Salmon
with Sautéed Greens
(page 178)

DAY 3

BREAKFAST
Oat Pancakes with Apple Compote (page 41)

SNACK
Herb Popcorn (page 73)

LUNCH
Salad with Sesame Garlic Dressing, Garlic Flatbread, grapes (pages 235, 104)

SNACK
Mango Coconut Smoothie (page 68)

DINNER
Fajita Chicken Rice Bowl (page 163)

DAY 4

BREAKFAST
Sweet Potato Ginger Muffins, butter or plant-based spread (page 54)

SNACK
Oat Crackers, mango (page 80)

LUNCH
Acorn Squash Soup, Oatmeal Roll (pages 111, 46)

SNACK
Macadamia Nut Crunch, apple (page 79)

DINNER
Pesto Penne with Asparagus, mixed greens (page 151)

DAY 5

BREAKFAST
Quick Oats with Berries, Chia & Maple Syrup (page 26)

SNACK
Blueberry Bars (page 213)

LUNCH
Loaded Greek Salad, Garlic Flatbread, melon of choice (pages 90, 104)

SNACK
Rice Cakes with Coconut Butter & Fruit (page 71)

DINNER
Oven-Fried Chicken, Onion Rings, Cauliflower Mash (pages 183, 142, 133)

DAY 6

BREAKFAST
Sweet Potato Hash with Fried Eggs (page 35)

SNACK
Deep Purple Smoothie (page 67)

LUNCH
Roasted Carrot & Garlic Hummus, Oat-Flour Wrap, Sweet & Savory Salad (pages 116, 100, 97)

SNACK
Macadamia Nut Crunch, melon of choice (page 79)

DINNER
Rosemary & Garlic Chicken Breasts with Vegetables (page 200)

DAY 11

BREAKFAST
Sweet Potato Ginger Muffins, butter or plant-based spread (page 54)

SNACK
Deep Purple Smoothie (page 67)

LUNCH
Mango Bean Salad, Corn Tortilla chips, melon of choice (pages 89, 101)

SNACK
Rice Cakes with Coconut Butter & Fruit (page 71)

DINNER
Zucchini Latkes with Applesauce, mixed greens (page 184)

DAY 12

BREAKFAST
Sweet Potato Hash with Fried Eggs (page 35)

SNACK
Apple Oatmeal Bars (page 51)

LUNCH
Carrot, Lentil & Kale Salad, Oatmeal Roll, grapes (pages 95, 46)

SNACK
Herb Popcorn, Melon Cooler (pages 73, 76)

DINNER
Asian Stir-Fry Noodles, Garlic Broccoli (pages 171, 124)

DAY 13

BREAKFAST
Maple Stovetop Donuts (page 39)

SNACK
Mango Coconut Smoothie (page 68)

LUNCH
Beet & Sweet Potato Rösti, grapes (page 98)

SNACK
Cherry Berry Sorbet (page 207)

DINNER
Lettuce-Wrapped Burgers, Caramelized Onions, Ketchup, Thyme Garlic Fries (pages 167, 191, 229)

DAY 14

BREAKFAST
Crepes with Blueberries & Whipped Cream (page 62)

SNACK
Macadamia Nut Crunch, apple (page 79)

LUNCH
Summer Succotash, Oat Crackers, melon of choice (pages 130, 80)

SNACK
Maple Popcorn, sliced veggies of choice (page 72)

DINNER
Spaghetti Squash with Chicken Meatballs & Pomodoro Sauce, mixed greens (page 192)

DAY 15

BREAKFAST
Maple Stovetop Donuts
(page 39)

SNACK
Blueberries & Cream
Smoothie Bowl
(page 31)

LUNCH
Summer Quinoa Salad,
mixed greens, apple
(page 109)

SNACK
Roasted Carrot & Garlic
Hummus, sliced veggies
of choice **(page 116)**

DINNER
Cod Cakes with Mango
Sauce, Super Salad with
Sesame Garlic Dressing
(pages 177, 86)

DAY 16

BREAKFAST
Sweet Potato Hash with
Fried Eggs **(page 35)**

SNACK
Oat Crackers, Whipped
Coconut Cream
(pages 80, 75)

LUNCH
Superfood Stew, Garlic
Flatbread, grapes
(pages 119, 104)

SNACK
White Bean & Basil Dip,
sliced veggies of choice
(page 85)

DINNER
Salmon Apple Salad,
Roasted Vegetables
(pages 175, 138)

DAY 17

BREAKFAST
Blueberry Corn Muffins,
butter or plant-based
spread **(page 52)**

SNACK
Mango Coconut
Smoothie **(page 68)**

LUNCH
Loaded Greek Salad,
Oatmeal Roll, melon of
choice **(pages 90, 46)**

SNACK
Maple Sugar Popcorn,
apple **(page 72)**

DINNER
Vegetable Coconut
Curry, mixed greens
(page 168)

DAY 18

BREAKFAST
Sweet Potato Ginger Muffin,
butter or plant-based spread
(page 54)

SNACK
Macadamia Nut Crunch,
apple **(page 79)**

LUNCH
Roasted Asparagus with
Fried Eggs & Pea Shoots,
Roasted Vegetables **(pages
92, 138)**

SNACK
Herb Popcorn, mango
(page 73)

DINNER
Black Bean Burgers,
Caramelized Onions,
Ketchup, Cucumber Dill
Salad **(pages 160, 191, 229, 127)**

DAY 23

BREAKFAST
Purple Sweet Potato
Donuts **(page 48)**

SNACK
Deep Purple Smoothie
(page 67)

LUNCH
Super Salad with
Sesame Garlic Dressing,
Oatmeal Roll
(pages 86, 46)

SNACK
Mango Bean Salad,
Corn Tortilla chips
(pages 89, 101)

DINNER
Fajita Chicken Rice Bowl
(page 163)

DAY 24

BREAKFAST
Quick Oats with Berries,
Chia & Maple Syrup
(page 26)

SNACK
Macadamia Nut Crunch,
apple **(page 79)**

LUNCH
Acorn Squash Soup,
Garlic Flatbread, grapes
(pages 111, 104)

SNACK
Herb Popcorn, fruit of
choice **(page 73)**

DINNER
Zucchini Noodles &
Chicken Scampi, mixed
greens with Caesar
Dressing
(pages 159, 226)

DAY 25

BREAKFAST
Vegetable Omelet, fruit
of choice **(page 36)**

SNACK
Roasted Carrot & Garlic
Hummus, sliced veggies
of choice **(page 116)**

LUNCH
Super Salad with Sesame
Garlic Dressing, Oatmeal
Roll **(pages 86, 46)**

SNACK
Mango Bean Salad,
Corn Tortilla chips
(pages 89, 101)

DINNER
Ginger Vegetable Fried
Rice with Sautéed Bok
Choy, Garlic Broccoli
(pages 188, 124)

DAY 26

BREAKFAST
Soft Ginger Granola,
milk of choice **(page 32)**

SNACK
apple, macadamia nuts
(whole or processed into
butter)

LUNCH
Summer Quinoa Salad,
mixed greens, fruit of
choice **(page 109)**

SNACK
Herb Popcorn, mango
(page 73)

DINNER
Grilled Chicken &
Vegetables **(page 156)**

DAY 19

BREAKFAST
Vegetable Omelet, fruit of choice (page 36)

SNACK
Blueberry Corn Muffin (page 52)

LUNCH
White Bean & Basil Dip, Oat-Flour Wrap, sliced veggies of choice, melon of choice (pages 85, 100)

SNACK
Deep Purple Smoothie (page 67)

DINNER
Salmon & Vegetable Medley (page 155)

DAY 20

BREAKFAST
Coconut Forbidden Rice Pudding (page 61)

SNACK
apple, pumpkin seeds (whole or processed into butter)

LUNCH
Kale & White Bean Soup, Oatmeal Roll, grapes (pages 115, 46)

SNACK
White Bean & Basil Dip, sliced veggies of choice (page 85)

DINNER
Vegetable Tart, Maple Thyme Carrots (pages 202, 134)

DAY 21

BREAKFAST
Purple Sweet Potato Donuts (page 48)

SNACK
Mango Coconut Smoothie (page 68)

LUNCH
Summer Quinoa Salad, mixed greens, fruit of choice (page 109)

SNACK
Macadamia Nut Crunch (page 79)

DINNER
Mushroom Rosemary Chicken, Cauliflower Mash, Rosemary Sea Salt Brussels Sprouts (pages 164, 133, 136)

DAY 22

BREAKFAST
Blueberries & Cream Smoothie Bowl (page 31)

SNACK
Melon Cooler (page 76)

LUNCH
Beets & Greens Salad, Oat Crackers, fruit of choice (pages 103, 80)

SNACK
Roasted Carrot & Garlic Hummus, sliced veggies of choice (page 116)

DINNER
Sesame Chicken, Garlic Broccoli (pages 194, 124)

DAY 27

BREAKFAST
Maple Scone, fruit of choice (page 56)

SNACK
Mango Coconut Smoothie (page 68)

LUNCH
Carrot, Lentil & Kale Salad, Garlic Flatbread (pages 95, 104)

SNACK
Oat Crackers, White Bean & Basil Dip (pages 80, 85)

DINNER
Mushroom Risotto, Roasted Vegetables (pages 186, 138)

DAY 28

BREAKFAST
Vegetable Omelet, Soft Oatmeal Bread (pages 36, 58)

SNACK
Maple Scone (page 56)

LUNCH
Loaded Greek Salad, apple (page 90)

SNACK
Macadamia Nut Crunch, fruit of choice (page 79)

DINNER
Beef Tenderloin with Herb Butter, Cauliflower Mash, asparagus (pages 196, 133)

DAY 29

BREAKFAST
Blueberry Corn Muffins, butter or plant-based spread (page 52)

SNACK
Fruit Plate with Whipped Coconut Cream (page 75)

LUNCH
Summer Quinoa Salad, mixed greens, fruit of choice (page 109)

SNACK
Herb Popcorn, sliced veggies of choice (page 73)

DINNER
Buddha Bowl with Sunflower Dressing, Butternut Squash with Brown Butter & Sage (pages 198, 141)

DAY 30

BREAKFAST
Sweet Potato Hash with Fried Eggs (page 35)

SNACK
apple, pumpkin seeds (whole or processed into butter)

LUNCH
Superfood Stew, Garlic Flatbread, fruit of choice (pages 119, 104)

SNACK
Oat Crackers, Roasted Carrot & Garlic Hummus (pages 80, 116)

DINNER
Mockaroni & Cheese, Sweet & Savory Salad (pages 172, 97)

Eating Out

Eating out can prove particularly difficult on a special diet. But you can go to restaurants and still maintain an anti-inflammatory and low-histamine diet. Keep these guidelines in mind.

MENTION UP FRONT THAT YOU HAVE A STOMACH CONDITION. Depending on your sensitivity level, you can say that you have an allergy to the foods that trigger your worst reactions.

TELL THE SERVER WHAT YOU *CAN* EAT. If you're not sure, it's always easier to focus on what you want rather than what you're avoiding. That way your server can point you to the appropriate dish(es).

FOR BREAKFAST, EGGS AND POTATOES ARE A SAFE BET. If they're not already on the menu, scrambled eggs with scallions, onions, or other low-histamine veggies are super easy for a cook to make. Another easy, tasty choice that's often available is oatmeal with berries and maple syrup or brown sugar.

AVOID CHEESE, BACON, AND SAUSAGE. They may sound delicious, but they're not worth the trouble.

ASK FOR VEGETABLES TO BE COOKED IN OLIVE OIL WITH FRESH HERBS AND A LITTLE SALT. Depending on your symptoms, have them throw in some garlic for additional flavor.

SALADS ALSO MAKE A GOOD, EASY OPTION. Again, avoid the cheese and croutons and go for lots and lots of veggies.

FOR THE DRESSING, REQUEST A WEDGE OF LEMON AND A SIDE OF OLIVE OIL. It's DIY, but you know exactly what you're getting.

AVOID BUFFETS. That food has been sitting there for a long time, allowing histamine to build up.

MENTION THAT YOU CAN EAT ONLY FRESH MEAT COOKED TO ORDER. Grilled salmon or chicken is an easy way to go.

MAKE SURE THE MEAT HASN'T BEEN MARINATED. It never hurts to ask.

POTATOES MAKE LOVELY SIDES. Sweet, roasted, or baked—yes, yes, yes.

AMERICAN RESTAURANTS ARE GREAT PLACES FOR A SAFE, BALANCED MEAL. You can order grilled steak, chicken, or fish with a baked potato or sweet potato and a side of veggies or a salad with olive oil and lemon juice for dressing.

MOST ITALIAN RESTAURANTS OFFER GLUTEN-FREE PASTA. Order it with chicken, broccoli, olive oil, and/or garlic. If you're eating at a rustic Italian restaurant, order grilled chicken with vegetables. Confirm that the mashed potatoes are made from scratch with just butter or milk.

FOR CHINESE OR THAI, YOU CAN'T GO WRONG WITH STIR-FRIED VEGETABLES. Request it with chicken, ginger, olive oil, and/or garlic and rice. Unmarinated grilled chicken skewers are a nice option at Thai restaurants. Veggie spring rolls in rice wrappers also could work, but ask about the filling.

BE CLEAR AND SPECIFIC. Say: "No soy sauce, fish sauce, or any sauces." If you know your worst triggers, mention them by name.

AVOID MARINADES, AGED MEATS OR OLD FISH, BROTHS, AND ALCOHOL. Ask when the restaurant takes delivery of their fish. Remember that restaurant broth can contain lots of histamine. Cooks often use alcohol in sauces.

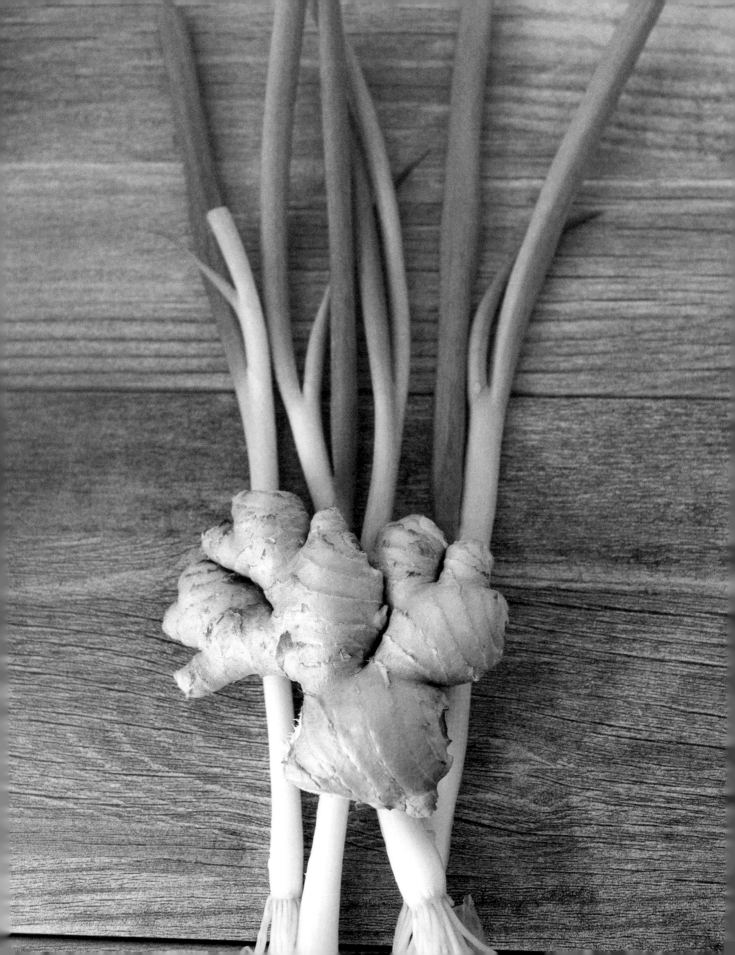

Holiday Menus

· ·

Holiday eating can feel like a minefield. What can you make that everyone will enjoy? What can you eat that won't trigger a reaction? Here's a selection of menu ideas that's great for all of the different holidays throughout the year. If you're eating at someone else's house, politely confirm that the food prep is low-histamine friendly—fresh ingredients that avoid store-bought broths and temperature-abused proteins. Better yet, ask the host nicely to make one or more recipes from this book!

Chinese New Year

- Asian Stir-Fry Noodles (page 171)
- Cherry Berry Sorbet (page 207)
- Garlic Broccoli (page 124)
- Ginger Vegetable Fried Rice with Sautéed Bok Choy (page 188)
- Sesame Chicken (page 194)

Passover

- Butternut Squash & Arugula Salad (page 112)
- Cherry Berry Sorbet (page 207)
- Grilled Chicken & Vegetables (page 156)
- Mango Cantaloupe Sorbet (page 220)
- Maple Thyme Carrots (page 134)
- Rosemary & Garlic Chicken Breasts with Vegetables (page 200)
- Rosemary Sea Salt Brussels Sprouts (page 136)
- Zucchini Latkes with Applesauce (page 184)
- Zucchini Noodles & Chicken Scampi (page 159)

Easter

- Blueberry Peach Galette (page 216)
- Carrot Apple Cupcakes (page 210)
- Coconut Lemon Bars (page 215)
- Cornmeal Waffle Egg Sandwiches (page 44)
- Fruit Tart with Mascarpone Cream (page 218)
- Roasted Asparagus with Fried Eggs & Pea Shoots (page 92)
- Vegetable Tart (page 202)

Summer Barbeque or Cookout

- Beef Tenderloin with Herb Butter (page 196)
- Black Bean Burgers (page 160)
- Blueberry Bars (page 213)
- Coconut Lemon Bars (page 215)
- Cucumber Dill Salad (page 127)
- Grilled Chicken & Vegetables (page 156)
- Lettuce-Wrapped Burgers (page 167)
- Loaded Greek Salad (page 90)
- Mango Bean Salad (page 89)
- Mango Cantaloupe Sorbet (page 220)
- Mango Salsa Salmon (page 149)
- Melon Cooler (page 76)
- Pesto Penne with Asparagus (page 151)
- Quinoa (Beet & Corn Salad (page 106)
- Salmon & Vegetable Medley (page 155)
- Summer Quinoa Salad (page 109)
- Summer Succotash (page 130)
- White Bean & Basil Dip (page 85)

Thanksgiving

- Acorn Squash Soup (page 111)
- Beet & Sweet Potato Rösti (page 98)
- Beets & Greens Salad (page 103)
- Blueberry Peach Galette (page 216)
- Butternut Squash & Arugula Salad (page 112)
- Butternut Squash with Brown Butter & Sage (page 141)
- Carrot Apple Cupcakes (page 210)
- Cauliflower Mash (page 133)
- Cranberry Chutney (page 228)
- Fall Harvest Salad (page 129)
- Fruit Tart with Mascarpone Cream (page 218)
- Lettuce-Wrapped Burgers (page 167)
- Maple Thyme Carrots (page 134)
- Mockaroni & Cheese (page 172)
- Roasted Vegetables (page 138)
- Rosemary Sea Salt Brussels Sprouts (page 136)
- Thyme Garlic Fries (page 145)

Hanukkah

- Acorn Squash Soup (page 111)
- Beet & Sweet Potato Rösti (page 98)
- Butternut Squash with Brown Butter & Sage (page 141)
- Fall Harvest Salad (page 129)
- Maple Stovetop Donuts (page 39)
- Roasted Asparagus with Fried Eggs & Pea Shoots (page 92)
- Shortbread Cookies (page 208)
- White Bean & Basil Dip (page 85)
- Zucchini Latkes with Applesauce (page 184)

Christmas

- Beef Tenderloin with Herb Butter (page 196)
- Beet & Sweet Potato Rosti (page 98)
- Beets & Greens Salad (page 103)
- Blueberry Peach Galette (page 216)
- Cauliflower Mash (page 133)
- Fruit Tart with Mascarpone Cream (page 218)
- Maple Scones (page 56)
- Maple Thyme Carrots (page 134)
- Oatmeal Rolls (page 46)
- Rosemary Sea Salt Brussel Sprouts (page 136)
- Shortbread Cookies (page 208)

Party Spread

- Apple Oatmeal Bars (page 51)
- Asian Stir-Fry Noodles (page 171)
- Blueberry Peach Galette (page 216)
- Caramelized Onion & Arugula Pizza (page 191)
- Carrot Apple Cupcakes (page 210)
- Coconut Lemon Bars (page 215)
- Corn Tortilla chips (page 101)
- Fruit Plate with Whipped Coconut Cream (page 75)
- Fruit Tart with Mascarpone Cream (page 218)
- Mango Salsa (page 230)
- Maple Sugar Popcorn (page 72)
- Oat Crackers (page 80)
- Onion Rings (page 142)
- Ranch Dressing (page 234)
- Roasted Carrot & Garlic Hummus (page 116)
- Shortbread Cookies (page 208)
- Thyme Garlic Fries (page 145)
- Vegetable Tart (page 202)
- White Bean & Basil Dip (page 85)

Reintroducing Foods

Research has shown that when adopting a low histamine anti-inflammatory diet, most people notice an improvement in their symptoms within about a month. Those with more severe cases of histamine intolerance, like MCAS, might benefit from spending more time on the diet, but you should start liberalizing the diet after a month to see what kind of histamine load your body can handle. Everyone has slightly different trigger foods and foods that unexpectedly don't cause any problems. Amount also matters. Keep a food diary as you reintroduce each new food. Try one new food—just one—every day. If you notice symptoms, repeat the new food the next day to confirm it was the food and not another factor. Try a small portion at first. You still want your diet to be anti-inflammatory, so increase plant-based foods first. Healthy foods are a must.

Here's the order in which you should consider reintroducing certain categories of foods to your diet.

1. Some fruits
Try bananas, your favorite stone fruits, some raspberries, strawberries, and dates. Still go easy on citrus and other dried fruits.

2. Avocados, tomatoes, and spinach
Avocado has high histamine levels, but it's also rich in nutrients, antioxidants, and good fats. Tomatoes and spinach also provide many phytonutrients and vitamins.

3. Tree nuts and oils
Reintroduce these as much as you can tolerate. They also contain valuable nutrients.

4. Dark chocolate
Chocolate contains flavonoids and antioxidants, and some people can handle it well in small amounts.

5. Dairy
Buttermilk, cottage cheese, feta cheese, sour cream, and yogurt are less problematic than aged cheeses. Adding these may increase your ability to tolerate more sauces and dressings, and a little sour cream on a fajita is such a treat. Still, keep dairy intake low to remain anti-inflammatory.

6. Apple cider vinegar, rice vinegar, or white vinegar
Most people can tolerate these better than balsamic vinegar, sherry vinegar, wine vinegar or other aged versions.

7. Wheat
If you enjoy wheat, try adding it back. Go for whole-grain foods.

8. Tofu
If you used to eat a lot of tofu, add it back in moderation and avoid soy sauce and fermented foods such as miso and kimchi.

9. Aged meats and cheeses
You should continue to focus on fresh meats and cheeses.

10. Processed foods
You may find that an otherwise anti-inflammatory and low-histamine diet allows you to enjoy small amounts of conventional condiments or alcohol. Be careful not to overdo it.

The Low-Histamine Lifestyle

· ·

The recipes in this book will help reduce inflammation and histamine intake in your diet, but there are other ways to reduce histamine-related symptoms. Here are five more ways to help your body.

1. REDUCE STRESS

Research has demonstrated that stress can increase inflammation and might influence the onset of allergies, autoimmunity diseases, infections, and other illnesses. Chronic and acute stress also increase the brain's release of histamine, which has a correlation with increased anxiety. Stress hormones activate mast cells to release histamine and inflammatory molecules.

Using stress reduction techniques can reduce your body's histamine levels and reduce inflammation levels. Helpful techniques include hypnotherapy, meditation, acupuncture, and yoga. Exercise is important for keeping your body healthy and managing stress levels, but high-intensity exercise can increase histamine levels, so try the following low-intensity exercises: biking, elliptical machine, light jogging, light weight lifting, vinyasa yoga, and walking.

2. LIMIT EXPOSURE TO EXTREME TEMPERATURES

Hot and cold temperatures also can affect histamine release in the body. High histamine levels can increase body temperature through the central nervous system and through the hypothalamus, our body's control center. That's why some people feel a rush of heat or redness in the face when eating high-histamine foods.

Try not to overheat in the summer. Stay near air-conditioning when the temperature is hot, and go outside during the cooler times of the day. Layer and bundle up in the winter. This point is especially important for people with MCAS or mastocytosis.

3. LIMIT SUN EXPOSURE

Studies have shown that people with sun-induced hives had elevated histamine levels, and direct sunlight increases the amount of histamine released from mast cells. Sunburned skin in particular causes an inflammatory cascade. Wear a healthy, mineral-based sunscreen and avoid exposure from 10:00 a.m. to 2:00 p.m. in the summer months.

4. BEWARE OF CHEMICALS

Many people with mast-cell conditions struggle with chemical sensitivity. Essential oils or perfumes can cause cringing, watering eyes, sinus congestion, headaches, and feeling faint. Choose shampoos, conditioners, and lotions with minimal chemicals and fragrances. Coconut oil, for example, makes a great natural moisturizer.

5. REDUCE ALLERGENS IN YOUR ENVIRONMENT

Environmental allergens also can increase histamine levels. HEPA filters often make a huge difference—just make sure to change them regularly. An allergist can administer an environmental allergy test as well. It's always best to know what your allergies may be and whether or how you can reduce or remove them from your environment.

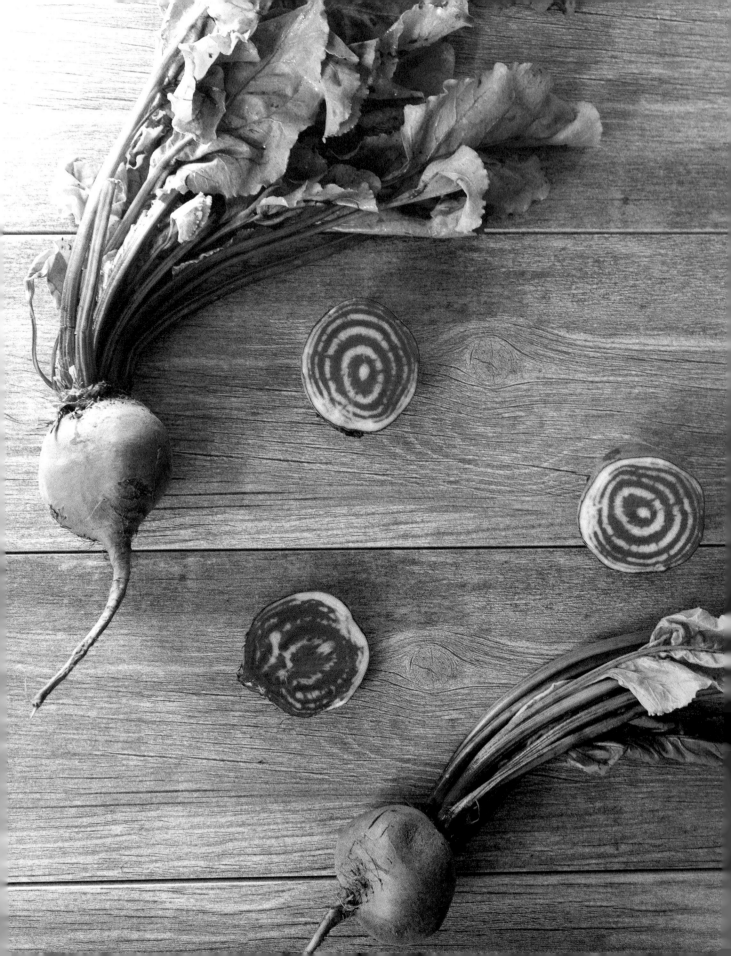

Acknowledgments

··

This book evolved as a project to help me focus on creating nutritional tools that could help others while I was experiencing devastating symptoms and a total upheaval in my diet and life. It was a form of creative therapy. Following a restrictive diet can feel so overwhelming even for a dietitian, so I set out to create recipes to guide myself and then others to a better path. Scientists still don't understand mast cell activation well, and increasing knowledge of this disorder and other associated histamine conditions remains very important.

My family always has been a huge support, and my parents always have pushed me to follow my dreams and never take no for an answer. Hard work will lead to rewards if you continue pushing ahead. I thank my husband, Eric, who was a huge support for this project, cleaning sinks full of dishes, tasting recipes that didn't come out so well, and watching the kids while I whipped up mountains of food. My sister, Kelsey, was a wonderful help as well on this project, editing the initial proposal before it was accepted for publication. My two sons, Henry and Zachary, continue to be my greatest inspiration and motivation for helping others and working to make the world a better place.

Special thanks to Sterling Publishing, James Jayo, and his team for publishing this fantastic nutrition cookbook, as I like to call it. Hopefully it will bring some welcome information and help to you and your family.

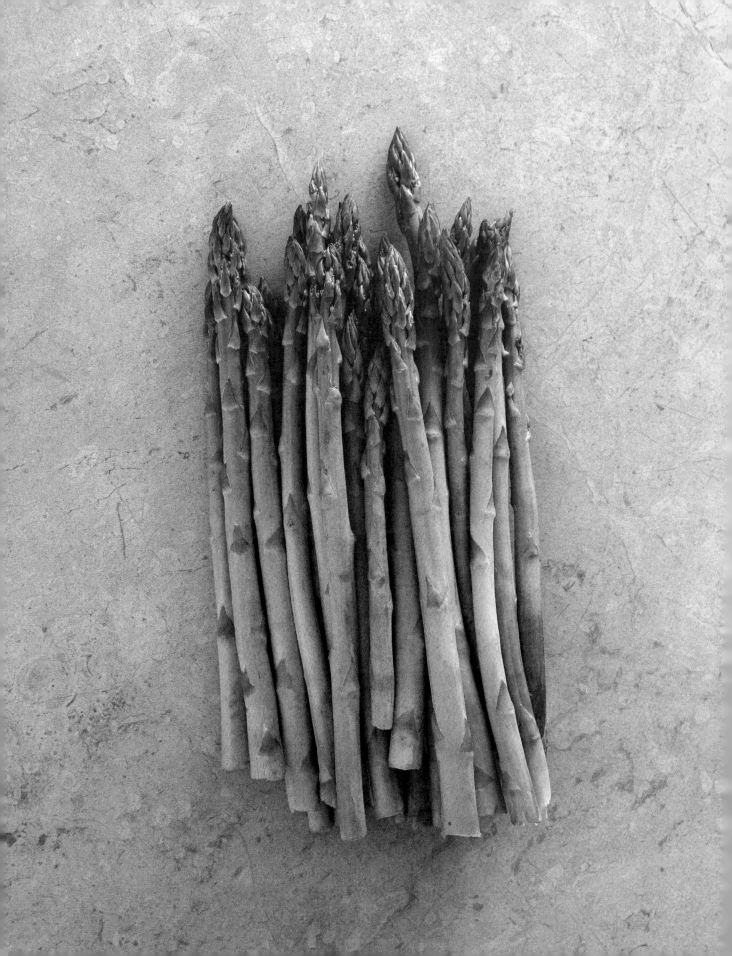

References

Ahui, M, Champy, P, et al. Ginger prevents Th2-mediated immune responses in a mouse model of airway inflammation. *International Immunopharmacology.* 2008; 8 (12): 1626–1632. https://www.ncbi.nlm.nih.gov/pubmed/18692598

Al-Khalaf, M. Thyme and thymol effects on induced bronchial asthma in mice. *Life Science Journal.* 2013; 10 (2). http://www.lifesciencesite.com/lsj/life1002/097_17864life1002_693_699.pdf

Al-Okbi, S. Nutraceuticals of anti-inflammatory activity as complementary therapy for rheumatoid arthritis. *Toxicology and Industrial Health.* 2012; 30 (8): 738–749. http://journals.sagepub.com/doi/abs/10.1177/0748233712462468.

Allergies. Life Extension.com. 2017. http://www.lifeextension.com/Protocols/Immune-Connective-Joint/Allergies/Page-refs

Arreola, R, et al. Immunomodulation and anti-inflammatory effects of garlic compounds. *Journal of Immunology Research.* 2015. https://www.hindawi.com/journals/jir/2015/401630/citations/

Barbara, G, Stanghellini, V, et al. Functional gastrointestinal disorders and mast cells: Implications for therapy. *Neurogastroenterology and Motility.* 2006; 18 (1): 6–17. https://www.ncbi.nlm.nih.gov/pubmed/16371078

Belch, J, Ansell, D, et al. Effects of altering dietary essential fatty acids on requirements for non-steroidal anti-inflammatory drugs in patients with rheumatoid arthritis: A double blind placebo controlled study. *Annals of the Rheumatic Diseases.* 1988; 47 (2): 96–104. http://ard.bmj.com/content/47/2/96.short

Bellik, Y, Boukraâ, L, et al. Molecular mechanism underlying anti-inflammatory and anti-allergic activities of phytochemicals: An update. *Molecules.* 2013; 18 (1): 322–353. http://www.mdpi.com/1420-3049/18/1/322

Bellik, Y, Hammoudi, S, et al. Phytochemicals to prevent inflammation and allergy. *Recent Patents on Inflammation and Allergy Drug Discovery.* 2012; 6. https://www.researchgate.net/profile/Yuva_Bellik/publication/221849962_Phytochemicals_to_Prevent_Inflammation_and_Allergy/links/547712150cf245eb43729c69/Phytochemicals-to-Prevent-Inflammation-and-Allergy.pdf

Bohn, L, Storsrud, S, et al. Self-reported food-releated gastrointestinal symptoms in IBS are common and associated with more severe symptoms and reduced quality of life. Am J Gastroenterol. 2013: 108(5):634–41. https://www.ncbi.nlm.nih.gov/pubmed/23644955

Buhner, S, Reese, I, et al. Pseudoallergic reactions in chronic urticaria are associated with altered gastroduodenal permeability. *Allergy*. 2004; 59 (10): 1118–1123. http://onlinelibrary.wiley.com/doi/10.1111/j.1398-9995.2004.00631.x/full

Capozzi, V, Russo, P, et al. Biogenic amines degradation by *Lactobacillus plantarum*: Toward a potential application in wine. *Frontiers in Microbiology*. 2012; 3: 122. https://www.ncbi.nlm.nih.gov/pmc/articles/PMC3316997/

Chakravarty, N. Inhibition of histamine release from mast cells by nigellone. *Annals of Allergy*. 1993; 70 (3): 237–242. http://europepmc.org/abstract/med/7680846

Chatzi, L, Apostolaki, G, et al. Protective effect of fruits, vegetables and the Mediterranean diet on asthma and allergies among children in Crete. *Thorax* 2007; 62 (8): 677–683. http://thorax.bmj.com/content/62/8/677.short

Chen, B, Wu, P, et al. Antiallergic potential on RBL-2H3 cells of some phenolic constituents of *Zingiber officinale* (ginger). *Journal of Natural Products*. 2009; 72 (5): 950–953. http://pubs.acs.org/doi/pdf/10.1021/np800555y

Choi, S, Kang, M, et al. Antiallergic activities of pigmented rice bran extracts in cell assays. *Journal of Food Science*. 2007; 72 (9): S719–S726. http://onlinelibrary.wiley.com/doi/10.1111/j.1750-3841.2007.00562.x/full

Cicerale, S, Lucas, L, Keast, R. Antimicrobial, antioxidant and anti-inflammatory phenolic activities in extra virgin olive oil. *Current Opinion in Biotechnology*. 2011; 23 (2): 129–135. https://www.researchgate.net/publication/51723160_Antimicrobial_antioxidant_and_anti-inflammatory_phenolic_activities_in_Extra_Virgin_OLive_Oil

Elenkov, L, Chrousos, G. Stress hormones, Th1/Th2 patterns, pro/anti-inflammatory cytokines and susceptibility to disease. *Trends in Endocrinology and Metabolism*. 1999; 10 (9): 359–368. http://www.sciencedirect.com/science/article/pii/S1043276099001885

Estruch, R. Anti-inflammatory effects of the Mediterranean diet: The experience of the PREDIMED study. *Proceedings of the Nutrition Society*. 2010; 69 (3): 333–340. https://www.cambridge.org/core/journals/proceedings-of-the-nutrition-society/article/antiinflammatory-effects-of-the-mediterranean-diet-the-experience-of-the-predimed-study/9DDD3527738A1E1E0EE8B0D0C9DE21F6/core-reader

Feldman, J. Histaminuria from histamine-rich foods. *Archives of Internal Medicine*. 1983; 143 (11): 2099–2102. http://jamanetwork.com/journals/jamainternalmedicine/article-abstract/603788

Finn, D, Walsh, J. Twenty-first century mast cell stabilizers. *British Journal of Pharmacology*. 2013; 170 (1): 23–37. https://www.ncbi.nlm.nih.gov/pmc/articles/PMC3764846/

Garcia Marcos, L, et al. Influence of Mediterranean diet on asthma in children: A systematic review and meta-analysis. 2013. *Pediatric Allergy and Immunology*. 2013; 24 (4): 330–338. http://onlinelibrary.wiley.com/doi/10.1111/pai.12071/full

Goda, H, Hoshino, K, et al. Constituents in watercress: Inhibitors of histamine release from RBL-2H3 cells induced by antigen stimulation. *Biological and Pharmaceutical Bulletin*. 1999; 22 (12): 1319–1326. https://www.ncbi.nlm.nih.gov/pubmed/10746164

Grazlottin, A, Skaper, S, Fusco, M. Mast cells in chronic inflammation, pelvic pain and depression in women. *Gynecological Endocrinology.* 2014; 30 (7): 472–477. http://www.tandfonline.com/doi/abs/10.3109/09513590.2014.911280

Grzanka, A, Machura, E, et al. Relationship between vitamin D status and the inflammatory state in patients with chronic spontaneous urticaria. *Journal of Inflammation.* 2014; 11: 2. https://journal-inflammation.biomedcentral.com/articles/10.1186/1476-9255-11-2

Guida, B, Martino, C, et al. Histamine plasma levels and elimination diet in chronic idiopathic urticaria. *European Journal of Clinical Nutrition.* 2000; 54: 155–158. https://www.researchgate.net/profile/Bruna_Guida2/publication/12620419_Histamine_plasma_levels_and_elimination_diet_in_chronic_idiopathic_urticaria/links/0912f50adcbb5ac5a7000000.pdf

Haugen, M, Fraser, D, Førre, Ø. Diet therapy for the patient with rheumatoid arthritis? *Rheumatology.* 1999; 38 (11): 1039–1044. https://academic.oup.com/rheumatology/article/38/11/1039/1783279/Diet-therapy-for-the-patient-with-rheumatoid

Hawk, J, et al. Elevated blood histamine levels and mast cell degranulation in solar urticaria. *British Journal of Clinical Pharmacology.* 1980; 9 (2): 183–186. http://onlinelibrary.wiley.com/doi/10.1111/j.1365-2125.1980.tb05831.x/full

Inoue, T, Sugimoto, Y, et al. Anti-allergic effect of flavonoid glycosides obtained from Mentha piperita L. *Biological Pharmacology Bulletin.* 2002; 25 (2): 256–259. https://www.ncbi.nlm.nih.gov/pubmed/11853178

Intahphuak, S, Khonsung, P, Panthong, A. Anti-inflammatory, analgesic, and antipyretic activities of virgin coconut oil. *Pharmaceutical Biology.* 2010; 48 (2): 151–157. http://www.tandfonline.com/doi/abs/10.3109/13880200903062614

Ito, C. The role of brain histamine in acute and chronic stresses. *Biomedicine and Pharmacotherapy.* 2000; 54 (5): 263–267. http://www.sciencedirect.com/science/article/pii/S0753332200800694

Izquierdo-Casas J, et al. Low serum diamine oxidase (DAO) activity levels in patients with migraine. *Journal of Physiology and Biochemistry.* 2018; 74 (1): 93–99. https://link.springer.com/article/10.1007/s13105-017-0571-3

Jarisch, R, Wantke, F. Wine and headache. *International Archives of Allergy and Immunology.* 1996; 110: 7–10. http://www.karger.com/Article/Abstract/237304

Joneja, J. Could It Be Histamine. 2013. http://www.foodsmatter.com/allergy_intolerance/histamine/articles/histamine_rose-08-13.html

Joneja, J. The histamine and tyramine restricted diet. Mastocytosis Society Canada. 2012. https://www.jillcarnahan.com/downloads/HistamineRestrictedDiet.pdf

Kahlson, G, Rosengren, E, Thunberg, R. Observations on the inhibition of histamine formation. *The Journal of Physiology.* 1963; 169 (3): 467–486. https://www.ncbi.nlm.nih.gov/pmc/articles/PMC1368714/pdf/jphysiol01211-0001.pdf

Kaiser, P, et al. Anti-allergic effects of herbal product from *Allium cepa* (bulb). *Journal of Medical Food.* 2009; 12 (2): 374–382. http://online.liebertpub.com/doi/abs/10.1089/jmf.2007.0642

Kalus, U, et al. Effect of *Nigella sativa* (black seed) on subjective feeling in patients with allergic diseases. *Phytotherapy Research.* 2003; 17 (10): 1209–1214. http://onlinelibrary.wiley.com/doi/10.1002/ptr.1356/full

Kang, O, Lee, J, Kwon, D. Apigenin inhibits release of inflammatory mediators by blocking the NF-kB activation pathways in the HMC-1 cells. *Immunopharmacology and Immunotoxicology.* 2010; 33 (3): 473–479. http://www.tandfonline.com/doi/abs/10.3109/08923973.2010.538851

Kanter, M, Coskun, O, H Uysal. The antioxidative and antihistaminic effect of *Nigella sativa* and its major constituent, thymoquinone, on ethanol-induced gastric mucosal damage. *Archives of Toxicology.* 2006; 80 (4): 217–224. https://link.springer.com/article/10.1007/s00204-005-0037-1

Katske, F, et al. Treatment of interstitial cystitis with a quercetin supplement. *Techniques in Urology.* 2001; 7 (1): 44–46. https://www.ncbi.nlm.nih.gov/pubmed/11272677

Khanna, R, MacDonald, J, Levesque, B. Peppermint oil for the treatment of irritable bowel syndrome: A systematic review and meta-analysis. *Journal of Clinical Gastroenterology.* 2014; 48 (6): 505–512. https://www.ncbi.nlm.nih.gov/pubmed/24100754

Komericki, P, Klein, G, et al. Histamine intolerance: Lack of reproducibility of single symptoms by oral provocation with histamine: A randomized, double-blind, placebo controlled cross-over study. *Wiener Klinische Wochenschrift.* 2011; 123 (1): 15–20. http://link.springer.com/article/10.1007/s00508-010-1506-y

Kovacova-Hanuskova, E, et al. Histamine, histamine intoxication and intolerance. *Allergologia et Immunopathologia (Madrid).* 2015; 43 (5): 498–506. https://www.ncbi.nlm.nih.gov/pubmed/26242570

Kremer, J, Lawrence, D, Petrillo, G, et al. Effects of high dose fish oil on rheumatoid arthritis after stopping nonsteroidal anti-inflammatory drugs. Clinical and immune correleates. Arthritis Rheum. 1995: 38(8):1107–14.

Kritas, S, et al. Mast cell involvement in rheumatoid arthritis. *Journal of Biological Regulators and Homeostatoc Agents.* 2013; 27 (3): 655–660. https://www.ncbi.nlm.nih.gov/pubmed/24152834

Lamprecht, H. Food Compatability List: Histamine. Swiss Interest Group Histamine Intolerance (SIGHI). Updated 2016. http://www.mastzellaktivierung.info/downloads/foodlist/21_FoodList_EN_alphabetic_withCateg.pdf

Lundius, E, et al. Histamine influences body temperature by acting on H1 and H3 receptors on distinct populations of preoptic neurons. *Journal of Neuroscience.* 2010; 30 (12): 4369–4381. https://www.ncbi.nlm.nih.gov/pmc/articles/PMC2853029/

Magerl, M, Pisarevskaja, D, et al. Effects of a pseudoallergen-free diet on chronic spontaneous urticaria: A prospective trial. *Allergy.* 2010; 65 (1): 78–83.

Maintz, L, Benfadal, S, et al. Evidence for a reduced histamine degradation capacity in a subgroup of patients with atopic eczema. *Journal of Allergy and Clinical Immunology.* 2006; 117 (5): 1106–1112. http://www.sciencedirect.com/science/article/pii/S009167490502600X

Maintz, L, Bieber, N, Novak, N. Histamine intolerance in clinical practice. *Deutsches Ärzteblatt.* 2006; 103 (51–52): 3477–3483. https://www.aerzteblatt.de/pdf/103/51/a3477e.pdf 26. Kahlson, G, Rosengren E, et al. The site of increased formation of histamine in the pregnant rat. *The Journal of Physiology.* 1958; 144 (2): 337–348. http://onlinelibrary.wiley.com/doi/10.1113/jphysiol.1958.sp006105/abstract

Maintz, L, Novak, N. Histamine and histamine intolerance. *American Journal of Clinical Nutrition* 2007; 85 (5): 1185–1196. http://ajcn.nutrition.org/content/85/5/1185.long

Masini, E, Bani, D, et al. Pea seedling histaminase as a novel therapeutic approach to anaphylactic and inflammatory disorders. *Scientific World Journal.* 2007; 7: 888–902. https://www.ncbi.nlm.nih.gov/pubmed/17619775

Min, S, Ryu, S, Kim, D. Anti-inflammatory effects of black rice, cyanidin-3-O-beta-D-glycoside, and its metabolites, cyanidin and protocatechuric acid. *International Immunopharmacology.* 2010; 10 (8): 959–966. https://www.ncbi.nlm.nih.gov/pubmed/20669401

Mizuguchi, D, Das, A, et al. Suppression of histamine signaling by probiotic Lac-B: A possible mechanism of its anti-allergic effect. *Journal of Pharmacological Science.* 2008; 107 (2): 159–166. https://www.ncbi.nlm.nih.gov/pubmed/18544899

Mueller, M, Hobiger, S, Jungbauer, A. Anti-inflammatory activity of extracts from fruits, herbs and spices. *Food Chemistry.* 2010; 122 (4): 987–996. http://www.sciencedirect.com/science/article/pii/S0308814610003158

Music, E, Korosec, P, et al. Serum diamine oxidase activity as a diagnostic test for histamine intolerance. *Wien Klin Wochenschr.* 2013; 125 (9–10): 239–243. http://www.ncbi.nlm.nih.gov/pubmed/23579881

Nagel, G, et al. Effect of diet on asthma and allergic sensitization in the International Study on Allergies and Asthma in Childhood (ISAAC) Phase Two. *Thorax.* 2010; 65 (6): 516–522. http://thorax.bmj.com/content/65/6/516?sid=

Nasri, S, Anoush, M, Narges, K. Evaluation of analgesic and anti-inflammatory effects of fresh onion juice in experimental animals. *African Journal of Pharmacy and Pharmacology.* 2012; 6 (23): 1679–1684. http://www.academicjournals.org/journal/AJPP/article-full-text-pdf/003A40229389

Nigrovic, P, Lee, D. Mast cells in inflammatory arthritis. *Arthritis Research and Therapy.* 2005; 7 (1): 1–11. https://www.ncbi.nlm.nih.gov/pmc/articles/PMC1064877/

Ning, Z, Hong, L, et al. Anti-inflammatory effect of curcumin on mast cell mediated allergic responses in ovalbumin-induced allergic rhinitis mouse. *Cellular Immunology.* 2015; 298 (1–2): 88–95. http://www.sciencedirect.com/science/article/pii/S0008874915300228

Nishio, A, Ishiguro, S, Miyao, N. Specific change of histamine metabolism in acute magnesium-deficient young rats. *Drug Nutrient Interactions.* 1987; 5 (2): 89–96. https://www.ncbi.nlm.nih.gov/pubmed/3111814#maincontent

Nugroho, A, Ikawati, Z, et al. Effects of benzylidenecyclopentanone analogues of curcumin on histamine release from mast cells. *Biological and Pharmaceutical Bulletin.* 2009; 32 (5): 842–849. https://www.ncbi.nlm.nih.gov/pubmed/19420752

O'Mahony, L. Host-microbiome interactions in health and disease. *Clinical Liver Disease.* 2015; 5 (6): 142–144. http://onlinelibrary.wiley.com/doi/10.1002/cld.484/full

Park, H, Lee, S, et al. Flavonoids inhibit histamine release and expression of pro-inflammatory cytokines in mast cells. *Archives of Pharmacal Research.* 2008; 31: 1303. http://link.springer.com/article/10.1007%2Fs12272-001-2110-5

Park, J. Identification and quantification of a major antioxidant and anti-inflammatory compound found in basil, lemon thyme, mint, oregano, rosemary, sage and thyme. *International Journal of Food Sciences and Nutrition.* 2011; 62 (6): 577–584. http://www.tandfonline.com/doi/abs/10.3109/09637486.2011.562882

Priyadarshani, W, Rakshit, S. Screening selected strains of probiotic lactic acid bacteria for their ability to produce biogenic amines (histamine and tyramine). *International Journal of Food Science and Technology.* 2011; 46 (10): 2062–2069. http://onlinelibrary.wiley.com/doi/10.1111/j.1365-2621.2011.02717.x/abstract

Reinhard, G, Lindmark, L, Frondoza, C. Ginger—An herbal medicinal product with broad anti-inflammatory actions. *Journal of Medical Food.* 2005; 8 (2): 125–132. http://online.liebertpub.com/doi/abs/10.1089/jmf.2005.8.125

Roschek Jr, B, et al. Nettle extract (*Urtica dioica*) affects key receptors and enzymes associated with allergic rhinitis. *Phytotherapy Research.* 2009; 23 (7): 920–926. http://onlinelibrary.wiley.com/doi/10.1002/ptr.2763/abstract

Rosell-Camps, A, et al. Histamine intolerance as a cause of digestive complaints in pediatric patients. *Scielo.* 2013; 105 (4). http://scielo.isciii.es/scielo.php?script=sci_arttext&pid=S1130-01082013000400004&lng=en&nrm=iso&tlng=en

Rudick, C, et al. Mast cell-derived histamine mediates cystitis pain. *PLOS ONE.* 2008; 3 (5): e2096. http://journals.plos.org/plosone/article/comments?id=10.1371/journal.pone.0002096

San Mauro Martin, I, Brachero, S, Garicano Vilar, E. Histamine intolerance and dietary management: A complete review. *Allergologia et Immunopathologia (Madrid).* 2016; 44: 475–483. http://www.elsevier.es/en-revista-allergologia-et-immunopathologia-105-articulo-histamine-intolerance-dietary-management-a-S0301054616300775#bib0260

Sant, G, Theoharides, T. The role of mast cell in interstitial cystitis. *Urologic Clinics of North America.* 1994; 21 (1):41–53. http://europepmc.org/abstract/med/8284844

Saurez, A, Feramisco, J, et al. Psychoneuroimmunology of psychological stress and atopic dermatitis: Pathophysiologic and therapeutic updates. *Acta Dermato-Venereolgica,* 2012; 92 (1): 7–18. http://www.ingentaconnect.com/content/mjl/adv/2012/00000092/00000001/art00003

Sears, B. Anti-inflammatory diets. *Journal of the American College of Nutrition.* 2015; 34 (1): 14–21. http://www.tandfonline.com/doi/abs/10.1080/07315724.2015.1080105

Sköldstam, L, Hagfors, L, Johansson, G. An experimental study of a Mediterranean diet intervention on patients with rheumatoid arthritis. *Annals of the Rheumatic Diseases.* 2003; 62 (3): 208–214. http://ard.bmj.com/content/62/3/208

Smolinska, S, Jutel, M, et al. Histamine and gut mucosal immune regulation. *European Journal of Allergy and Clinical Immunology.* 2014; 69 (3): 273–281. http://onlinelibrary.wiley.com/doi/10.1111/all.12330/full

Sridevi, G, Gopkumar, P, et al. Pharmacological basis for antianaphylactic, antihistaminic and mast cell stabilization activity of ocimum sanctum. *Internet Journal of Pharmacology.* 2008; 7 (1). http://ispub.com/IJPHARM/7/1/6038

Thomas, C, Hong, T, et al. Histamine derived from probiotic *Lactobacillus reuteri* suppresses TNF via modulation of PKA and ERK signaling. *PLOS ONE* 2012; 7 (2): e31951. http://journals.plos.org/plosone/article?id=10.1371/journal.pone.0031951

Vysakh, A, et al. Polyphenolics isolated from virgin coconut oil inhibits adjuvant induced arthritis in rates through antioxidant and anti-inflammatory action. *International Immunopharmacology*. 2014; 20 (1): 124–130. http://www.sciencedirect.com/science/article/pii/S1567576914000800

Wagner, N, Dirk, D, et al. A Popular myth—low-histamine diet improves chronic spontaneous urticaria—fact or fiction? *Journal of the European Academy of Dermatology and Venereology*. 2016. Accessed online 12/1/2016. http://onlinelibrary.wiley.com/doi/10.1111/jdv.13966/full

Wang, X, Wujiang, L et al. Evidence for the role of mast cells in cystitis-associated lower urinary tract dysfunction: A multidisciplinary approach to the study of chronic pelvic pain research network animal model study. *PLOS ONE*. 2016. http://journals.plos.org/plosone/article?id=10.1371/journal.pone.0168772

Wantke, F, Gotz, M, et al. Histamine-free diet: treatment of choice for histamine-induced food intolerance and supporting treatment for chronic headaches. *Clinical and Experimental Allergy*. 1993; 23 (12): 982–985. http://onlinelibrary.wiley.com/doi/10.1111/j.1365-2222.1993.tb00287.x/full

Watanabe, J, Shinmoto, H, Tsushida, T. Coumarin and flavone derivatives from estragon and thyme as inhibitors of chemical mediator release from RBL-2H3 cells. *Bioscience, Biotechnology, Biochemistry*. 2005; 69 (1): 1–6. https://www.jstage.jst.go.jp/article/bbb/69/1/69_1_1/_pdf

Weng, Z, Zhang, B, et al. Quercetin is more effective than cromolyn in blocking human mast cell cytokine release and inhibits contact dermatitis and photosensitivity in humans. *PLOS ONE*. 2012; 7 (3): e33805. http://journals.plos.org/plosone/article?id=10.1371/journal.pone.0033805

Worm, M, Fiedler, E, et al. Exogenous histamine aggravates eczema in a subgroup of patients with atopic dermatitis. *Acta Dermato-Venereologica*. 2009; 89 (1): 52–56. http://www.ingentaconnect.com/content/mjl/adv/2009/00000089/00000001/art00010

Yoon, J, Baek, S. Molecular targets of dietary polyphenols with anti-inflammatory properties. *Yonsei Medical Journal*. 2005; 46 (5): 585–596. https://synapse.koreamed.org/search.php?where=aview&id=10.3349/ymj.2005.46.5.585&code=0069YMJ&vmode=FULL

Zaeem, Z, Zhou, L, Dilli, E. Headaches: A review of the role of dietary factors. *Current Neurology and Neuroscience Reports*. 2016; 16: 101. https://link.springer.com/article/10.1007/s11910-016-0702-1

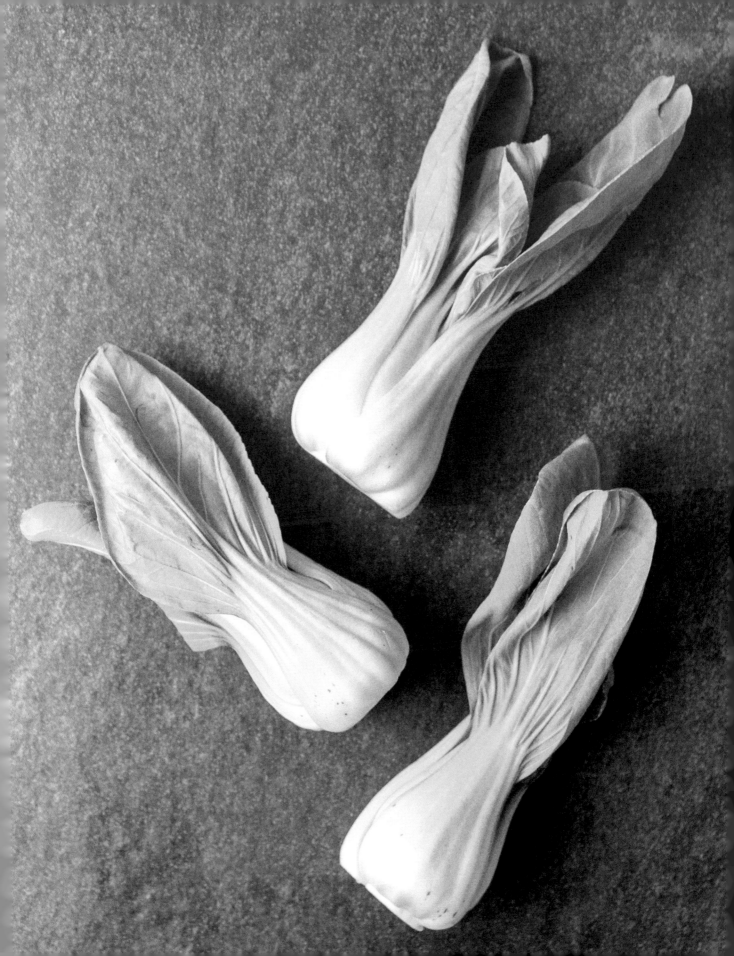

Index

....

Note: Page numbers in *italics* include photos of recipes.